doris inc.

doris inc.

A Business Approach to Caring
for Your Elderly Parents

SHIRLEY ROBERTS

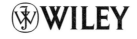

John Wiley & Sons Canada, Ltd.

Library and Archives Canada Cataloguing in Publication Data

Roberts, Shirley, 1951-
   Doris Inc. : a business approach to caring for your elderly parents / Shirley A. Roberts.

Includes index.
ISBN 978-1-118-10022-6

   1. Aging parents—Care. 2. Adult children of aging parents—Family relationships. I. Title.

HQ1063.6.R61 2011   306.874084'6   C2011-902467-5

ISBN 978-1-11810165-0 (ePDF); 978-1-11810163-6 (eMobi); 978-1-11810164-3 (ePUB)

Production Credits
Cover design: Adrian So
Interior text design: Thomson Digital
Typesetter: Thomson Digital
Printer: Trigraphik | LBF

John Wiley & Sons Canada, Ltd.
6045 Freemont Blvd.
Mississauga, Ontario
L5R 4J3

Printed in Canada
1 2 3 4 5 LBF TRI 16 15 14 13 12

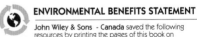

ENVIRONMENTAL BENEFITS STATEMENT

John Wiley & Sons - Canada saved the following resources by printing the pages of this book on chlorine free paper made with 100% post-consumer waste.

TREES	WATER	ENERGY	SOLID WASTE	GREENHOUSE GASES
49	47,570	76	6,013	15,631
FULLY GROWN	GALLONS	MILLION BTUs	POUNDS	POUNDS

Environmental impact estimates were made using the Environmental Paper Network Paper Calculator. For more information visit www.papercalculator.org.

Contents

Acknowledgments

Doris Inc., the venture, had a committed team to take care of my mother. Doris Inc., the book, also had a devoted team of people who gave generously of their time and talent to move this initiative forward, to read chapters in their area of expertise, and provide feedback. They all believe in my cause of empowering caregivers and improving the quality of life of elders. Like me, they also want readers to have accurate and practical information. I would like to wholeheartedly thank each and every one of them.

Physicians

Dr. Roger Wong, Clinical Professor of Geriatric Medicine, University of British Columbia; Head, Geriatric Consultation Program, Vancouver General Hospital

Dr. Tiffany Chow, Senior Clinician-Scientist, Rotman Research Institute; Assistant Professor, University of Toronto Neurology and Geriatric Psychiatry

Dr. Michael Chambers, family physician

Dr. Conrad Rusnak, family physician

Registered Nurses

Kathi Colwell, Program Manager, Physical Medicine and Rehabilitation, Providence Care, Kingston, Ontario

Margie Colbourne, Clinical Educator – Medicine, Western Health Care Hospital, Corner Brook, Newfoundland

Ina Taylor, ER nurse, Western Health Care Hospital, Corner Brook, Newfoundland

Linda Walker, life-care planner

Svea Murray, formerly director of nursing, working in nursing homes and hospice palliative care

Sue Epp, retired head nurse, formerly with Helen Henderson Care Centre

Other Eldercare Experts

Barb Thompson, retired nurse, formerly with the Alzheimer Society of Kingston, Ontario

Joyce Gordon, President and C.E.O, Parkinson Society Canada

Derek Mercey, Publisher, *The Care Guide*

Joel Coté, formerly senior manager, communications, South East Community Care Access Centre

Nancy Solomon, Director of Communications, Ontario Retirement Communities Association

Elaine Frost, President, Trusted Transitions, certified professional consultant on aging

Wendy Glass, retired nursing home admissions and marketing director

Financial Advisors

David Roberts, C.A. and Investment Advisor, BMO Nesbitt Burns, my brother and partner in Doris Inc.

Alan Riccardi, Manager, Estate and Trust Administration, MD Private Trust Company

Nick Cagna, accountant, Cagna and Associates

Other Professionals

Doug Walker, lawyer focusing on estate law

Henry Wong, Vice-President and Creative Director, Tenzing Communications

Christine Lasky, Vice-President Strategic Initiatives, Princess Margaret Hospital Foundation

Barbara Galli, Ph.D., author and research scholar, Faculty of Religious Studies, McGill University

Gary McCracken, President, McCracken & Partners Executive Search Inc. and former board member, Alzheimer Society of Toronto

Literary Experts

John Wiley & Sons' publishing team, especially Jennifer Smith, Alison Maclean, and Leah Fairbank

Rick Broadhead of Rick Broadhead & Associates, my literary agent

Stacey Cameron, freelance editor

Caregivers

Ella Hillier

Sue Milne

Family

Mitch Fenton, my beloved husband, in-home editor, and sounding board

Grace Wilson, my cousin and a caregiver

Lorne Taylor, my cousin

Introduction

It is my true honour and pleasure to be invited to write the introduction to *Doris Inc.* This book is certainly more than a useful resource for individuals who provide care to seniors, but is also a true and touching story of how we can survive and be successful in providing the best possible care to our loved ones.

I am especially impressed with how *Doris Inc.* is written in a systematic and easy-to-understand manner. Let's face it, providing care for seniors is a complex endeavour that can be difficult to capture in simple words. The topics and information presented here are relevant and current. The recommendations are practical and with appropriate attention to details. This step-by-step guide will help families complete the various tasks that are important in looking after seniors. The Top Tips at the end of each chapter help to cover the salient take-home messages. This book is a handy resource for seniors and for those who already or will soon be caring for them.

Doris Inc. includes very specific help for families facing the challenge of dementia. Recent data from the study entitled *Rising Tide: The Impact of Dementia on Canadian Society* released by the Alzheimer Society reveals alarming new statistics about the projected economic and social costs of dementia in Canada. Findings from this national study indicate that if nothing changes over the next 30 years, the prevalence of dementia will more than double from 2008 figures to an estimated 1.1 million Canadians[1]. Over this time frame, the associated economic burden is projected to reach a cumulative total of over $870 billion[2]. The relevance and timeliness of *Doris Inc.* is self-evident.

Traditionally, physicians and other health-care professionals have always played the role of health advocates on behalf of their patients in the provision of care, especially for those with dementia, who have more difficulty speaking for themselves. *Doris Inc.* offers a road map for family care providers to collaborate with health-care teams, and in doing so, will advance the health and well-being of older individuals, their communities, and the general population.

Congratulations to Shirley Roberts and her team of eldercare experts who helped to ensure the accuracy of the information provided. I believe this book will be an important addition to the resources available to support seniors and those who provide care for them.

—Roger Y.M. Wong, BMSc, MD, FRCPC, FACP
Clinical Professor of Geriactric Medicine
Assistant Dean, Postgraduate Medical Education
Faculty of Medicine, University of British Columbia
Head, Geriatric Consultation Program
Vancouver General Hospital

---

[1] *Rising Tide: The Impact of Dementia on Canadian Society.* Alzheimer Society, 2009
[2] Ibid.

1

My Heart-Wrenching Caregiving Dilemma

Early in the 20th century, Lamaline, Newfoundland, was a bustling fishing village at the bottom of the boot-shaped Burin Peninsula. Life was tough back then. The only connections with the outside world were telegrams and the coastal boats that brought mail, household essentials, and fishing supplies.

Apart from a district nurse, and Granny Foote and Granny Crocker who assisted women with giving birth, medical help was a rough 25-mile ride by horse-drawn box cart or sleigh to the town of Grand Bank. Antibiotics hadn't been discovered yet, so many villagers died from infections and a lack of emergency medical care before they reached their senior years.

Lamaline was a close-knit community of families whose ancestors had come from England, and the elderly were an integral part. The Bonnells, the Cakes, the Collins, the Footes, and the Haskells were some of the big families, but the Hilliers were the largest clan of all. Brightly painted fishing sheds and wooden houses that decorated the settlement reflected the lively spirit of the people, and none more so than that of my mother, Doris Hillier.

Doris was born on September 8, 1918, the fourth of Daniel and Amelia Hillier's six children. She was a happy and energetic child whose entire face would light up and her brown eyes would twinkle whenever she smiled. Her enthusiastic expression of delight continued until she reached the ripe old age of 90.

In 1921, Doris' older brother Aubrey died at the age of six of the croup, a common childhood respiratory infection. Death knocked on my mother's own door four years later, at the age of seven, when she contracted scarlet fever. Her burial dress was ready and waiting, but miraculously she survived with a hearing loss and a heart murmur. Although she recovered some hearing in her right ear, she remained deaf in her left due to a perforated eardrum, an impairment for which she was bullied at school.

Back then there was no organized care or training for people with special needs, and hearing aids were neither affordable nor readily available. Fortunately, her father had been a schoolteacher and he tutored her during her illness and then helped her when she couldn't hear lessons in class. Doris soon learned to lip-read and later, with the help of hearing aids in both ears, she never let her hearing impairment hold her back from anything she wanted to do.

In 1929, the Lamaline villagers were confronted with a situation that tested their ability to overcome adversity. On November 18, at 5:02 p.m., a 7.2-magnitude earthquake shook the Grand Banks, about 250 kilometres south of the Burin Peninsula. It was felt as far away as New York, Montreal, and Portugal, and was the sixth-largest earthquake ever recorded in Canada.

My Aunt Gladys, one of Mom's two sisters, described how at 7:30 p.m. she watched the ocean mysteriously and eerily recede from the shore to expose the ocean floor. A few minutes later, villagers in more than 40 outports along the foot of the peninsula were terrified when they saw a gigantic white foamy wall of salt water coming toward them. Able-bodied residents ran to higher ground. Three successive waves crashed over the land, crushing whatever was in their way and rising as high as 42 feet in the long narrow bays.

The devastating tsunami killed 28 people, mostly women, children, and the elderly, in six communities between Port au Bras and Lamaline. Villagers would never forget that clear moonlit night when they stood helpless, watching houses float away with kerosene lamps still burning brightly, until the ocean completely swallowed the buildings with their family or neighbours inside. Many traumatized survivors were left with only the shirts on their backs after their homes and winter provisions were destroyed. My grandparents' house was located on low-lying ground just a road and a meadow away from the ocean. The dwelling sustained serious flood damage, but the family was spared. From that day forward my mother was frightened of the ocean and never learned to swim.

The Burin Peninsula recovered, a testament to how families, neighbours, and their beloved district nurse, Dorothy Cherry, rallied to assist one another during a crisis. The homeless received shelter, food, and warm clothing from neighbours or relatives, and Nurse Cherry travelled by horseback and on foot to the worst-hit communities to attend to the injured and sick. Able-bodied men rebuilt the homes once aid arrived from the Newfoundland, Canadian, American, and British governments, and from public donations.

In this same resourceful way, a sisterhood of village women supported their parents and other elderly residents. Seniors' lives were intertwined with their large extended families and neighbours. Nursing homes didn't exist in this remote part of the country, and the hospital was too far away, so seniors typically lived and died in their own homes, surrounded by their loved ones.

Retaining the values she learned growing up, Doris became a caring and resourceful young woman with a passion for life. She had a positive attitude and always found the best in people and in situations. Doris' quick wit and ability to see the lighter side of life made her fun to be with.

In 1936, following in the footsteps of many young people from fishing villages, Doris moved to St. John's at the age of 18. While there she met Ed Roberts, a handsome man in his late 20s. He was born in 1911, in the pretty fishing village of Brigus on the shore of Conception Bay, 50 miles from St. John's.

Matchmakers say opposites attract and that was certainly the case for outgoing Doris and shy and serious Ed. However, in the mid-1940s, Doris made the gutsy decision to move to Toronto in search of more plentiful jobs, as her sister Gladys and her family had done. Ed missed his girlfriend so much that he pulled up stakes in St. John's and moved to Toronto. On August 14, 1947, Doris and Ed, aged 29 and 36, were married. My brother David was born in 1948 and I came along three years later.

In the fifties, women of my mother's generation often stayed at home to care for their children, and later in life brought their elderly parents into their home to care for them, until they needed hospitalization in their final days. My grandfathers both died in their late 60s, but my grandmothers lived until their mid-90s. They were very well cared for at home by my aunts in Corner Brook and St. John's, Newfoundland.

When I was seven, my parents built a small cottage in the Kawarthas, not far from Campbellford, Ontario, on the Crowe River. Over time, other Newfoundlanders, mostly from Lamaline and Taylor's Bay, came to "the Crowe" to build cottages. These were happy family times, filled with great friendships, lots of swimming and boating, and evening card games that my mother loved.

Eventually, David and I grew up, graduated from the Ivey School of Business at the University of Western Ontario, and started our business careers, his in accounting and mine in marketing. Our parents sold their family home in Toronto and retired to Cobourg, a charming town on Lake Ontario, about 60 miles east of Toronto. They adjusted well to retirement and grew attached to the town and their small brick bungalow. Mom quickly made new friends, often inviting them over for tea, homemade date squares, and a chat. By this time, she took great pleasure in the small things in life, especially in conversations with her family, neighbours, and friends.

Mom finally got her driver's licence in her early 60s, but she seldom drove because Dad was afraid she wouldn't hear cars around her well enough to avoid dangerous situations. The drive to the cottage became increasingly stressful as Dad gradually lost his nerve to drive beyond Cobourg or at night. By then Mom had also lost her nerve to get behind the wheel. When my father turned 76 and my mother 69, they realized that they could no longer keep their cottage and grounds in tip-top shape as they had always done. My parents reluctantly decided to sell their beloved cottage. What they hadn't yet realized was that they were also bidding farewell to the active era of their retirement years. This had been a carefree period unencumbered by time, work, and parenting responsibilities, and unrestricted by their physical and mental capabilities.

As Doris and Ed transitioned into their 80s, it was evident that their bodies were wearing out and they had both lost some of their mental sharpness. They would, on occasion, purposefully walk into a room and then forget why they went there. They would also lose keys or important documents and have to spend frantic moments searching for them. My mother managed all the family finances and was proud that she could complete annual income tax returns. Eventually, this task stressed her out so I helped collect the information to send to David, our family financial advisor, so that he could complete the return.

My parents progressively became less energetic. They stopped going to church regularly and watched it on TV instead. Their physical stature had noticeably shrunk, their hair thinned, and their eyesight and hearing worsened. Doris had maintained her shapely figure, but her spine formed the letter C, a sign of osteoporosis. She walked with a cane in her late 70s, but with increased frailty she used a walker more often to get around.

Sadly, on September 15, 2002, three weeks before his 91st birthday, my father died and my pillar of dependability instantly vanished. Family had come first in my father's life and he had always been there for us. There were times when knowing this made all the difference in dealing with life's challenges. Dad died of congestive heart failure after two trips to the Cobourg hospital emergency department, once in June and once two weeks before his death. I was with him in his final hours of consciousness and I'm so glad I was able to say to him, "you have been just the best father." He heard me and responded, "That's nice."

I was forced to bury my grief for my father because I immediately became my frail mother's primary caregiver, a strange new role for which I was ill prepared. I did the best I could to help her cope with this dramatic change in her life. We spoke every day on the phone, and I drove from Toronto to Cobourg every other Saturday to spend the day with her. I also hired help to do household chores, including cleaning the house, cutting the grass, and shovelling the snow, and I was in touch with her neighbours who volunteered to look in on her regularly.

I found Sue, a good Samaritan to the elderly, who became particularly fond of my mother. She took Mom grocery shopping and to medical appointments, stopped in for tea, and helped with the gardening. I thought at the time that I had all my bases covered. Doris was by nature very sociable so I expected that, after a reasonable period of time for mourning, she would be happy to move to a retirement residence where she could enjoy life once again with new friends, unencumbered by her house.

Meanwhile, I ran my marketing company, keeping clients happy by working five to six days a week at a hectic pace. I also tried to find time for Mitch, the lovely man in my life. It soon became very evident, however, that both Mom and her house were being sadly neglected. On one of my visits, I discovered unopened mail collecting dust, laundry lying in piles on her basement floor, a burnt-out hallway light bulb, expired milk and yogurt cluttering her fridge, and her blouse covered in tea stains. As I left that day, tears welled up in her eyes and in mine; it was painfully obvious to me that I wasn't keeping up. Nevertheless, I had no more time to devote to my mother, without giving up some essential aspect of my own life. I grasped the magnitude of my heart-wrenching dilemma with frustration, overwhelming sadness, and guilt.

I must confess I never expected to find myself in this predicament. Frankly, the subject of my parents' death and my own mortality stayed buried in my subconscious. When I *did* think about it, I imagined that we would die in our sleep one day after a wonderfully long and healthy life. The possibility of having to take care of my elderly parents, then later my spouse, and one day needing care myself never crossed my radar screen. Then it dawned on me just how naive I had been, and that I should have been better prepared for this task.

At the time, I hadn't realized that the social skills and activity levels of many seniors diminish greatly as they age, and they can become very reclusive once their spouse dies. Supplemental daily support and companionship are often needed by people in their 80s and 90s, whether they live on their own, in a retirement residence, or in a nursing home. They can become totally dependent upon other people for social interaction, mental stimulation, and activities that interest them. Compassionate deeds by kind souls are extremely important, because they give seniors a sense of belonging and create a diversion from their diminishing health and loneliness.

Mom definitely needed a lot more attention than I could give her to lessen her feelings of isolation. During that difficult transition period I noticed that when she had company or received a hug, her whole face would light up and the old familiar twinkle in her eyes returned.

Within two months of my father's death, my mother's grief was compounded by symptoms of Alzheimer's disease that surprisingly started to surface. At the time, I attributed her deep depression to the loss of her husband of 55 years, and to the stress of the change to her way of life. However, I was puzzled when I started to receive several calls a day from Mom fretfully asking the same question over and over again. I became even more alarmed when her neighbours and the parish nurse expressed their concern that "your mother is very confused and it isn't safe for her to be living on her own."

Now that I understand this debilitating brain disorder much better, I can recall the telltale signs of my mother's dementia symptoms: her forgetfulness, uncharacteristic irritability, episodes of anxiety and confusion, and withdrawal from her usual activities. She had rapidly lost her ability to live independently, and because David lived on the West Coast, her well-being became my responsibility.

For a year and a half, I helped my mother live as independently as she could, and I tackled her health and loneliness issues using what I call a solo firefighter approach to caregiving, focusing only on Mom's crisis of the day. Lacking the time and insight to organize a better solution made this an extremely stressful and sometimes insane period in my life. My efforts to take good care of Mom failed miserably, and I witnessed first-hand how our society's current method of caregiving can result in neglected seniors and burnt-out caregivers. I believe this is a result of socio-economic and demographic changes and medical advances that are rendering our current caregiving model obsolete.

Caregiving has become much more challenging for the baby-boom generation than it was for previous generations for a number of reasons. Typically, women take on the responsibility for eldercare; however, this custom is outdated because more female caregivers, the majority of whom are between the ages of 45 and 64, have demanding full-time jobs. Because more of these women went to college or university than in past generations, many had children later in life, who are more likely to still live at home when an elderly parent needs support.

Baby boomers also have a higher divorce rate, so caregivers today are more likely to be a single parent who bears household and care responsibilities alone. Families are typically smaller and more spread out today than they were in past generations. Caregivers often don't have relatives living nearby on whom they can rely. In our more transient society, we are more likely to be caring for a parent who lives in a different city, or even very far away.

Medical advances are extending the lives of our moms and dads but not eliminating chronic debilitating diseases that afflict the elderly, such as osteoporosis, Alzheimer's, or Parkinson's disease. More adult sons and daughters will, therefore, be responsible for a dependent parent, and will have caregiving duties for 5 to 10 years, or longer.

Our current caregiving approach works well for seniors who have immediate family willing to sacrifice their lives for them, a large extended family willing to help, or who have the financial resources to pay for the very best full-time care. However, many frail seniors live in an environment cut off from the rest of society, alone in their own home all day while their children work, or alone in a seniors' residence or nursing home. For these many neglected poor souls, our current caregiving approach simply doesn't work.

A staff member at a nursing home confessed to me one day that some families visit residents only once a month, some visit weekly but only for an hour, and still others don't even show up for birthdays or Christmas. Isolation and neglect is getting worse, because a scarcity of time and long-distance caregiving makes frequent visits impossible for many adult children. There are, however, other reasons for this lack of attention.

Some adult children mistakenly assume that the staff in retirement residences and nursing homes can fulfill all of their parents' needs, making their attentive care unnecessary. Others, especially men, don't really know what their caregiving role is, or they don't want to know, because they get squeamish helping their parent do things such as go to the bathroom. Frequently, sons and daughters are so absorbed in their own busy lives that they don't recognize when their parents need help. They may also be uncomfortable dealing with elderly parents who remind them of their own inevitable demise, or they have a feeling of futility in making much effort because there is no hope for recovery. I have often heard people admit that they infrequently visit Alzheimer's residents because, "my mother doesn't recognize me and I can't deal with that." Still other children, and even spouses, unconsciously resent their loved one getting sick and leaving them with the burden of care, and so can't face being with them often.

I knew my mother and I couldn't survive another year with her living in her own home so, after much coaxing, I convinced her to spend January in a retirement residence to see if she liked it. I think the thought of walking down cozy warm corridors rather than sliding on snow- and ice-laden roads enticed her to give this safer haven a fair chance. She moved back home in February, however, because she missed her house and neighbours so much, and threatened to never return to the retirement residence. Realizing Mom's resistance, I set about doing what was in her best interest, and that was convincing her to move to a safer environment, given her advancing dementia symptoms and the challenges of living by herself.

I patiently listened to her concerns, I asked her about her jovial new friend, Betty, who had taken her under her wing at the retirement residence, and I gently nudged her toward the best decision. By the end of March, after time to weigh retirement-residence life against living alone, Mom finally agreed to sell her house. This taught me an important lesson: that seniors, like all of us, need time to adjust to any change in their lives.

By June 2003, Mom's house had been sold and David came from Vancouver to move her into a retirement residence in Cobourg. Doris chose an apartment next door to Betty on the second floor where the residents' smoky-coloured Persian cat lived. One late summer afternoon, I was thrilled to hear my mother's laughter fill the hallway outside of Betty's apartment, as she and her new pal tried to hide their indulgence in a hot toddy. The duo soon became so inseparable that I nicknamed them "Frick and Frack." I was hopeful Mom would flourish with new friends and interests, and would live out the rest of her life in relative happiness with visits from me every two weeks. I felt optimistic because life was pretty good once again for Mom, David, Mitch, and me.

When I took a short break from my caregiving duties in the fall, Mom's situation seemed very much under control. Life stood still for a magical moment on September 26 when, surrounded by friends and relatives, Mitch and I got married. My mother was in her glory partaking in the festivities with her sister, her nieces and nephews, and lifetime friends.

Sadly, this would be the last large family gathering in which she would know who they all were. Our period of relative calm was very short lived. On December 23, my mother fell and broke her leg close to her hip, and spent three lonely months in the hospital because her brittle femur was so slow to heal.

Doris couldn't return to her retirement residence because her needs exceeded the level of care available. She had rapidly progressed to the middle stage of Alzheimer's disease and couldn't walk or propel her wheelchair. The hospital discharge planner told me that Mom needed to move to a nursing home. My mother dreaded the thought of ever living in an old-folks' home and we dreaded the thought of moving her there, because we heard stories of nursing staff neglect in the news. Unfortunately, we soon learned that we had no other option.

By this point, I urgently needed to find a better approach to caregiving because I was spending as much time putting out fires for Mom as I was consulting. Her quality of life and mine had taken serious nosedives ever since she landed in the hospital, and my caregiving duties would continue to increase as my mother became more dependent on me for her health and well-being.

In early April 2004, Doris moved into a new long-term care facility that was going through growing pains. The staff had never worked together before; indeed, some of the employees had never even worked in a nursing home. On my very first visit, a young and inexperienced personal support worker left my mother on the toilet unattended, got busy with another resident, and then totally forgot her.

Frantically, I went looking for staff to help, because my mother couldn't put any weight on her left leg, and I couldn't lift her back into her wheelchair on my own. I expected that at any moment she would fall on the floor and break yet another bone. I must have looked visibly upset, because the registered practical nurse called the administrator, who came running to calm me down and solve the problem. I never saw that personal support worker at the nursing home again.

The first Saturday in June was a beautiful warm, cloudless sunny day. After a very busy workweek, I was driving along the highway on my way to visit Mom as I did most Saturdays. My mind was churning a mile a minute. I wanted to spend this glorious day golfing with Mitch, but I needed to spend the day with my mother. As I neared my destination, I began to accept the reality that my duty that day was with Mom.

Over the past month, I'd noticed that Doris was not adjusting well to nursing-home life, and that a common and irreversible cycle had started. Dementia had taken a stronger hold of her behaviour and her social skills were fading noticeably. My mother was hesitant to strike up a conversation with passersby or attend social activities. She had made new friends in the retirement

residence, but not here, and she lacked the initiative to amuse herself by reading, listening to music, or watching her favourite TV
programs. Sadly, Doris was spending most of her days by herself
in her room and becoming depressed and despondent.

At times, even her room seemed like a scary unfamiliar
place, because she was losing her ability to speak for herself
when she needed help. She became easily distracted by other
people around her and lacked the focus to eat on her own. When
coaxed, she would eat, but it would take her a full hour to finish a
meal. Personal support workers couldn't stay with her that long,
because they had other residents to help, so Doris slowly started
to lose weight.

Residents in Doris' nursing home receive 20 minutes of personal one-on-one time from an activities coordinator each day,
and there are scheduled daily activities that they can participate
in, if someone takes them. These initiatives certainly help when
they are available, but they can't give residents the same quality
of life that they had when they lived with their families.

Many residents often fall asleep in their chair during the day
due to sheer boredom. Even Doris noticed how drowsy her peers
were during lunch one day when she glanced over at the next
table of residents in the dining room and said, "They're not so
lively over there." This took me totally by surprise because she
had been very quiet that morning. Her words sent me into a fit
of laughter.

When I arrived at the nursing home, I put on my happy face
to greet my mother. It is only human nature to want a cheerful
visitor, but this is especially important for a person with dementia. I learned through trial and error that Mom would echo my
moods. If I exhibited signs of being upset, she would become
upset too. I gave her a kiss and a gentle hug and read to her from
her favourite prayer book, which seemed to comfort her.

I helped Mom eat lunch and then took her outside for some
fresh air. At 2:30 p.m., I asked two personal support workers if
they could put my mother to bed for an afternoon nap. When
Doris laid her head on her pillow, she looked up to see that it was
one of her favourite personal support workers tucking her in.

With typical charm from her younger years she said, "Do you want to lie down with me?" The personal support worker was flattered at Doris' attempt to befriend her. She gave her a wide grin and said she would love to join her because she was very tired, but had far too much work to do. At that moment, for the very first time, I saw loneliness not only in my mother's eyes but also in her actions. I knew she missed my father terribly and also her family life and she no longer had a home to call her own. An hour later with great anguish I bid farewell to my mother and reluctantly headed back to Toronto.

As I drove home I felt torn between my conflicting roles. I needed to find more time for Mom, but I also needed to earn a living, and I wanted to spend more time with my new husband. I came to the depressing conclusion that the word *enough* isn't in the caregiver dictionary. I hadn't even hit the heavy lifting of late-life caregiving, let alone the enormous weight of palliative care, and already I couldn't hold my own.

Doris was lonely and I could never be with her enough to keep her happy. She wasn't eating well and I couldn't help her eat at every meal. Suddenly, a groundswell of feelings came over me. I worried that if I got burnt out and sick I would not be able to help my mother, and she would be even more abandoned. I felt my life had been put on hold and that made me very angry. I felt resentful of my brother who lived so far away, and whose life wasn't on hold. At the same time, I felt guilty that I resented him and that when my mother needed me the most I had let her down. I also felt helpless watching old age ravage my mother's frail body, because I knew I had no way to stop her decline.

I arrived back in Toronto mentally and physically tired, as I usually did after a day with my mother. To my surprise, despite feeling tormented my normal tenacity returned. My mind was overflowing with thoughts of how I could solve my crisis. I knew that David would be a willing partner in any scheme that would allow us to take better care of our mother. With great enthusiasm, I realized that it was within my power to find a way for my mother and me to suffer less.

To find a way to take better care of Mom and still have a life of my own, David and I instinctively drew upon our business experience and applied business disciplines to caregiving. We created a loving home environment with professional, attentive, and compassionate care for our elderly mother.

We used only our parents' middle-class financial resources, government-funded pensions and health-care support, and our determination. Mitch affectionately called our venture Doris Inc. because it resembled a business, and we have stuck with that name ever since. The driving force behind Doris Inc. was the endless love that David and I had for our one customer, our mother.

We noticed early on that our mother was happier and more comfortable than she was before we started Doris Inc., and by focusing on her capabilities rather than limitations, we enabled her to function as well as she could. My stress level was lower, and I had more free time, so my life was no longer on hold.

Our venture ran for five years, and although our mother's care needs became much more complex in the final stage of Alzheimer's disease, her life had been as good as it could have been every step along the way. At the same time, our new approach to caregiving gave me more personal time, including time to write key segments of this book, so that other caregivers and elders will hopefully have better lives together.

TOP TIPS

A Solo Firefighter Approach to Caregiving Doesn't Work

- Getting involved in caregiving only in emergency situations results in neglected loved ones, stressed out caregivers, and poor decisions.
- Caregiving is too big a job for one person. Caregivers need backup when they get sick and when they need a break.

Be Prepared

- Learning about eldercare before an aging parent or spouse needs your help will prepare you for the challenges that lie ahead.

Patience is a Virtue

- Seniors need time to adjust to any change in their life.

Home is Sweet Home

- Create a loving home environment for your aging parent, even if they can no longer live in their own home.

Keep them Busy

- Daily activities and companionship give seniors a sense of belonging, and create a diversion from their illnesses and loneliness.

Where There's a Will There's a Way

- Focus on a senior's capabilities, not their disabilities.

2

Creating Doris Inc. to Take Better Care of Mom and Me

Doris Inc. began with a conversation I had with my mother while she convalesced in the hospital. She said she found her days dreadfully long, there was nothing for her to do, and she was feeling very lonely and isolated. She asked if I could find someone to visit her regularly.

I felt bad that I lived 100 kilometres away and couldn't spend more time with Mom so I found a volunteer to visit her. High-school students in the area are required to complete community service to graduate; however, the teenager only came five times. I needed a more business-like approach: a broader search to find the right type of support, and a financial incentive to obtain the best-qualified people and continuity of care.

A massage therapist I had hired to treat Mom's broken leg recommended Sharon, a mother of four girls, who needed to make some extra money. We hired her to visit Mom in the hospital and once she moved into a nursing home. She turned out to be a godsend. A tremendously compassionate and thoughtful person, she had a gift for anticipating my mother's needs before anyone else did. Doris and her new companion bonded. Mom became more talkative and was returning to her old self again.

Sharon occasionally brought her daughters as well as their two affectionate kittens, which delighted my mother. Mom had better days when she had caring visitors who understood her well and tended to her needs. The value of outside help became increasingly apparent to me as her mental and physical health deteriorated.

The next challenge facing my brother and me was to create a loving home environment with the best professional health and personal care for our mother, without giving up our own independent lives. We drew upon our business experience and applied a tried-and-true business model to caregiving: leadership and operations.

Although Doris Inc. wasn't a real business, it possessed all the components of a well-run company: unified, proactive, and decisive family-care leadership, a well-coordinated care-team operation, clearly defined goals, and prudent financial management. We found that organizing our resources in this way worked best for the business of caregiving for elderly people. The chart on page 22 lays it out visually.

As family-care leaders, David and I got involved and diligently managed all aspects of our mother's care and well-being. Our first step was to carefully assess Mom's medical and physical requirements, as well as her social, emotional, intellectual, and spiritual ones. Our second step was to assemble a care-team operation, consisting of three care groups to provide the expertise and support necessary to meet all of her needs.

Our family caregiving team of David and me was responsible for ensuring that all of Mom's needs and wishes were met, because we knew her best. Our health-care team was responsible for our mother's medical, nutritional, and hygiene care. Her nursing home had good leadership; competent, compassionate, and dedicated nursing staff; a good family doctor who visited residents once or twice a week; and physiotherapists. Since Doris was wheelchair bound, we hired a massage therapist to augment the physiotherapy and a registered nurse who specialized in footcare. We also had a service-oriented audiologist who kept Mom's hearing aids in good repair.

As our mother's medical needs changed over the years, we requested referrals from her family doctor to an ear, nose, and throat specialist to clean the wax out of her ears, to a dermatologist to treat a pre-cancerous growth on her temple, and to an oral surgeon to remove infected roots of teeth that had fallen out. When Mom was in the hospital we worked with the hospital-care team that was assigned to her.

Our team of caregiver-companions were responsible for Mom's happiness and comfort and for helping her to eat. Mom's friend Sue, Sharon, and three more women whom we hired were her first caregiver-companions. As our mother descended into the middle stage of Alzheimer's disease, we hired retired personal support workers who had a wealth of professional experience helping frail seniors with their personal care, and they understood dementia well.

Clearly, life had changed since David and I formed Doris Inc., as you see in the table on page 22. Prior to this, my solo firefighter approach to caring for Mom had been crisis-driven with no backup plan in case I got sick or needed a break. I made hasty decisions without the benefit of good information and advice. As her health deteriorated, the number of emergencies increased, making life chaotic, stressful, and unpredictable for me.

Life wasn't great for Mom either. Her three-month hospital stay left her more anxious and confused than before. The hurried and intense care she received from health-care professionals and me was reactive to her latest crisis, and therefore lacking in empathy and patience. We certainly didn't work as a team, and there was little thought given to preventing future problems.

Family-care leadership and care-team operations were the two fundamentals of the Doris Inc. caregiving approach that brought calmness to our family. I felt empowered and in control. Our care teams worked collaboratively in the trenches to anticipate and meet all of Doris' needs as her health declined. I no longer worried all the time about Mom because she was receiving attentively good care, and my stress level was no longer off the Richter scale.

Doris Inc.'s Caregiving Approach

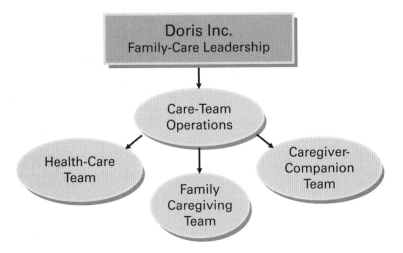

Difference in Caregiving Approaches

Solo Firefighter	Family-Care Leadership & Care-Team Operations
Approach	
• Crisis-driven • Little input into medical care • No backup • Hasty, ill-informed decisions made • Focus only on meeting physical needs	• Organized and proactive leadership • Care teams work collaboratively • Depth of resources • Time to make informed decisions • Focus on meeting physical, social, emotional, intellectual, and spiritual needs
End Result	
• Poorer decisions and care • Chaotic and stressful for everyone • More wasted time	• Attentively good care, no gaps or neglect • Peace of mind • Time-efficient care, fewer fires to fight

FAMILY-CARE LEADERSHIP

Family caregivers tend to passively give in to the dictates of the health-care system. When this happens, seniors and their families have little say in determining their own destiny. If there is no family-care leadership, aging loved ones, who have complex health issues in their final years, may become a low priority in health-care production lines. Family members need to demonstrate dedicated and passionate leadership, so that health-care professionals will be more likely to go the extra mile required to properly care for their mother, father, or spouse.

Even though David lives in Vancouver we became equal partners at the helm of Doris Inc. He and I agreed that we would always make decisions about Mom's care together. We demonstrated our unified voice when problems were brought to our attention, as well as when we discovered issues on our own. If hospital or nursing home staff, or a caregiver-companion received conflicting directions from us, it would have been more difficult for them to execute our mother's care effectively. Far too often families can't agree on an aging parent's care, resulting in fiery disputes between siblings over where their parent or parents should live, who should provide care, which doctor should be used, what specific medical treatment they should be given or denied, and how their care should be paid for.

Good information and advice from medical and eldercare experts leads to good decisions, strong leadership, and family harmony. Knowledgeable family caregivers feel more in control and less stressed. David and I actively made it our business to learn about Mom's medical conditions, medications, available support services, and the way hospitals and long-term care facilities operate. We learned how our health-care and caregiver-companion teams like to work, and treated them as part of our extended family by getting to know them personally. This ensured not only that our questions, concerns, and requests were realistic and well grounded, and therefore more likely to be addressed, but also that we made the best decisions we could for Mom.

Successful, well-run companies have a clear vision of what they want to accomplish, so setting goals is one of the C.E.O.'s most important roles. This practice makes great sense for family-care leaders, so that spouses, sons, and daughters jointly articulate the type of care and quality of life they want to provide. After lengthy discussions, David and I committed to achieve the following goals:

- give our mother professional and attentive care, delivered in a loving and comfortable home-like environment that met all of her needs;

- strongly advocate for our mother when issues related to her health were not being resolved quickly, or not in a way that we believed she would have wanted for herself, or that were not in her best interest; and

- carefully manage our mother's financial affairs, and spend her money wisely to fulfill her every need and desire for the rest of her life—and we agreed to pay for her expenses out of our own pockets if she ran out of money.

Defining roles and responsibilities is critical in the business of eldercare so that tasks are clear and allocated among family leaders, care teams, and individual care-team members, thus eliminating gaps and duplication. Jokingly, I told people that David was in charge of making money to run Doris Inc., and I was in charge of spending it. Of course, our leadership duties were more complex than that. David was in charge of Mom's financial affairs, a role he could fulfill from Vancouver. I was in charge of operations and advocacy.

I found my leadership responsibility quite daunting at times, especially when we had tough decisions to make, such as whether or not to put Mom through surgery to replace a pacemaker battery. I appreciated David's help so that I didn't have to play God on my own. On decisions that caused the most anguish, David and I searched for more information and advice. We thought about what Mom would have wanted for herself, we openly discussed the risks and rewards of each option, and then patiently made a decision together. Doris Inc. actually strengthened our relationship.

The culture of an organization is established by the standards, beliefs, attitudes, and actions of its leadership team, and can have a significant influence on a company's performance. In a healthy culture, employees understand their role in accomplishing goals, feel respected and valued by their leaders, and feel motivated to meet the standards of performance expected of them. David and I were persistent in our efforts to give our mother the very best care we could, and the care teams that we assembled clearly understood our goals and respected our actions. Our love and compassion for our mother fostered a Doris-centred culture for Doris Inc.

When my mother was younger she became a wise confidant to David and me, and to her nieces and friends. She shared insights to help us see the issues we were facing more clearly. One of her favourite pearls of wisdom was, "Feeling gratitude and not expressing it is like wrapping a present and not giving it," which was written by William Arthur Ward, an author, educator, and motivational speaker. She believed strongly in that motto and never forgot to thank people for their acts of kindness.

I was well schooled in her philosophy and expressed my heartfelt praise, respect, and gratitude to our health-care and caregiver-companion team members whenever they demonstrated initiative and dedication. For instance, I sent a well-deserved thank-you letter to Mom's doctor who, while he was on vacation, consulted with her cardiologist and called me with their opinion concerning the replacement of Doris' pacemaker battery. Christmas was the perfect occasion to formally express our gratitude with cards and gifts of thanks to those who took good care of Mom, as well as a small bonus for our caregiver-companions.

CARE-TEAM OPERATIONS

Doris Inc.'s care-team operations ran like the proverbial well-oiled machine. We had clearly defined roles and responsibilities, communication tools that fostered teamwork, and an effective monitoring and proactive problem-solving procedure.

As a key member of Doris Inc.'s family caregiving team, I spent three to four hours once a week caring for my mother, fulfilling the duties of a caregiver-companion. Mom and I found activities to enjoy together, such as having lunch, going outside to watch birds and admire the gardens, and attending nursing-home activities such as entertainment events, bazaars, and tea parties on Mother's Day.

On this level Doris Inc. served me as well, because these happy times helped me hold on to our mother-daughter relationship for as long as I could. I learned to appreciate every precious moment I spent pampering my mother, knowing that our days together were numbered. I enjoyed giving her hugs and kisses. I knew that she treasured those moments too because she usually closed her eyes for each embrace. I was also Doris Inc.'s head shopper, which I loved; indeed, I mimicked a doting new parent, searching for flattering outfits and accessories so Mom would never look frumpy.

My brother took on caregiving tasks that could be done from afar, such as working with the audiologist to repair or replace Mom's hearing aids when needed, and taking over caregiving when I went on vacation or travelled for business. He called in more frequently from Vancouver when I was away to see if there were any problems that required his attention. He usually came to visit Mom twice a year, and I took that time off.

Our caregiver-companion team had specific duties. In their role as a caregiver, they were responsible for helping Doris eat, brushing her hair and teeth, washing and moisturizing her face and hands, cleaning her eyeglasses, and replacing her hearing-aid batteries when she could no longer perform these activities of daily living on her own. Under the guidance of the nursing home's physiotherapist, they were to give her massages and help her stretch and do exercises that moved her arms and legs . They also found ways to make my mother more comfortable, such as putting a sweater or blanket on her when she was cool. Our caregiver-companions were also responsible for asking the nursing home's personal support workers to take Doris to the bathroom, to the spa for a bath, and to put her into bed after lunch for a nap and in the evening, if they hadn't already done so.

In their role as a companion, Mom's caregiver-companions were responsible for helping to meet her social, emotional, intellectual, and spiritual needs with conversation, hugs, playing her favourite music, and reading aloud. They also walked her around the nursing home for a change of scenery, or outside for some fresh air when the weather was warm and sunny. Her ladies took her to religious ceremonies that she enjoyed, and made arrangements with an activities coordinator to take her to entertainment and musical events.

Each caregiver-companion found their own way to pamper Doris and boost her self-esteem. One of them was also named Doris so we called her Doris II for fun. She loved to select Mom's clothes for the next day, complete with costume jewellery, as well as style her hair and apply her makeup. Jenny made neck pillows so Doris could nap in her wheelchair, and asked a friend to knit two shrugs, which resemble shawls with sleeves. Eleanor was great at getting Doris to stretch her muscles and joints, and often gave her a massage and a manicure, complete with nail polish. Joan loved to sing to Mom and Sharon cut her hair, played games, and continued to bring her girls to visit Doris once in a while.

We were blessed to have such caring people filling Mom's life with joy; indeed, they brought joy to me too when I saw my mother's glowing smile as they greeted her. This confirmed to me that I had chosen her caregiver-companions well.

Good people are the heart of any successful business and I learned through experience to find out what was in the heart of a prospective employee. I could teach a person their job, but I couldn't teach them good values. In the same way, I assessed doctors, nursing staff, and our caregiver-companions by the values I thought they held. When I hired new caregiver-companions, I looked for women whose family was a priority in their life, and who demonstrated that they had a big heart, through volunteer work or helping seniors in their own family. Mom was always present at the interviews, so I was able to look for women who showed a strong interest in her, interacted well with her, and seemed to have an innate ability to make her feel comfortable. Of course, she had to like them too. Despite her advancing Alzheimer's disease, I could tell when Mom didn't like a new caregiver-companion, personal support worker, or nurse. She would look concerned, pull away, and not eat well. Through trial and error, I learned that she liked gentle, soft-spoken women who were patient with her.

The caregiver-companions who worked out the best were primarily motivated to take the job because they had a passion to assist seniors, not simply because they needed the money. Ideally, they wanted to work part-time, and weren't looking for a full-time job, which would have been too disruptive for my mother when they left and a waste of time and money training them. The best employees lived no more than a 20-minute drive from the nursing home, so working two-hour shifts would be worth their while and winter road conditions wouldn't be as hazardous.

Retired personal support workers were the best caregiver-companions because they had the most experience with seniors who had chronic and debilitating diseases, and had more free time and flexibility. For them, taking care of Mom added meaning to their lives, making our arrangement a win-win situation.

Some candidates were referred to me by the parish nurse at Mom's church or by our other caregiver-companions. I also placed a help-wanted ad in the local community newspaper's classified section, which read: "Helper and companion wanted for lady in nursing home. Flexible, part-time hours. Retired PSW (Personal Support Worker) ideal." By hiring my caregiver-companions privately, rather than through an agency, I controlled the selection process, their duties, and had direct contact with them. It was also less expensive. Agencies at the time would have charged me $20 to $25 an hour, compared to the $14 that I paid our caregiver-companions directly. If I lived in another province or country or needed caregiver-companions on a temporary or emergency basis after Mom was convalescing from surgery, for example, then hiring care through an agency would have been a very welcomed alternative.

Unfortunately, not every caregiver-companion worked out. About a month after I hired one particular caregiver-companion, I discovered that she made Doris feel very uncomfortable. When this person worked a shift, my mother would glance up worriedly at her favourite nurse, whom she trusted. By this stage of Alzheimer's disease, Mom couldn't talk, but her body language and her big brown eyes expressed a cry for help. The nurse gave me all the details and conveyed her concern, so I quickly replaced the employee. In another case, a newly hired caregiver-companion on her very first shift spent 20 minutes on her cellphone while she was supposed to be assisting Doris eat her lunch. A personal support worker got the message to me about the incident and I let the individual go.

I scheduled 19 two-hour shifts a week around my mothers' meal times to provide help and companionship during the hours when she was most alert. Since Doris attended planned nursing-home activities, socialized with other residents, napped in the afternoon, and usually went to bed by 8:00 p.m., I didn't see the need to run shifts any longer. On the weekends, I only scheduled lunch and dinner shifts, so the personal support workers in Mom's nursing home unit helped her eat breakfast.

Frail elders with chronic and debilitating diseases can benefit from the care and attention of caregiver-companions, as can their primary family caregivers. Even if they can only afford a person for one hour a day, or two hours three times a week at a cost of $5,000 to $7,000 a year, or find volunteers to come when they can, it is well worth it. The senior's life will be enriched and their illnesses won't seem so burdensome to them.

Five caregiver-companions was the right number to handle 19 visits a week. I wanted them to look forward to the time that they spent with my mother. I felt that if they had a shift every day their job could have become an obligation rather than a pleasure, and put too many restrictions on their personal time.

Eleanor, Doris II, Jenny, Joan, and Sharon worked well as a team. They loved the flexibility of working the hours that best fit their personal schedules, and willingly covered for each other when someone went on holiday, was sick, or had an appointment.

Sharon or Eleanor, our caregiver-companions with the most seniority, trained new caregiver-companions and accompanied Doris to external medical appointments with specialists.

I had two strict rules for our caregiver-companions. First, they couldn't come to work if they had or suspected that they were getting a cold, flu, or anything that might be contagious. Viruses can spread like wildfire among vulnerable nursing-home residents with sometimes tragic results. If there is such an outbreak, the provincial Ministry of Health can order a lockdown of the facility or units within it, which means that visitors can't enter the locked-down unit until all residents have recovered.

The second rule was that our caregiver-companions, David, and I could administer care only to Doris. One day, Sharon tried to help a resident who was choking and turned blue. A registered practical nurse quickly arrived to take over from her. After that incident, the administrator made it clear that only the nursing staff were permitted to provide care to the other residents, because only they were covered by the long-term care facility's liability insurance.

Our workers had a common purpose in caring for Doris and they often exchanged ideas on the phone or over coffee about what worked best. Jenny surprised us with her dedication. While feeding Doris lunch one Sunday, she had a heart attack and was rushed by air ambulance to a hospital in Kingston. When she arrived, she insisted that her son call Sharon to find a replacement for her dinner shift that same day. Six weeks later, after a quadruple bypass, she was back working for Doris again. A year later, she was diagnosed with breast cancer, yet she insisted on doing her scheduled weekend shifts in between her chemotherapy treatments.

When mistakes are made in business, poor communications are often the cause. Good communications are even more important in caregiving because there are typically many people involved in an elder's care, as their diseases become more complex in their final years.

I created a communications tool called Doris' visitor book, which helped ensure a well-coordinated care operation between our caregiver-companions and me. I got the idea from a counsellor at the Alzheimer Society who recommended the chronicle because people with dementia can't always remember who came to visit them. Doris' friends learned that her visitor book was kept in the top drawer of her night table so they would post a note about their visit each time they came. Its main function was, however, as a caregivers' daily logbook of my mother's health status, comfort level, food and fluid intake, and any new problems so that we could carry on where the others left off. This was especially valuable when any of us had been away for a week. The logbook also provided David and me with an attendance record, because notations were made for every shift in chronological order, which was important when I hired a new caregiver-companion.

I gave our caregiver-companions guidelines about what notations we should highlight. For instance, if we had a new concern that we asked a registered practical nurse about, such as when I first noticed Doris' ankles starting to swell, we were to write down and highlight the question and the response. This allowed us to avoid asking the same question repeatedly. In this case, the registered practical nurse asked us to elevate Doris' feet when she lay down. If any of us received other instructions from the nursing staff, we recorded that as well.

Tracking lessons learned is important for business, and is particularly appropriate for caregiving. If our caregiver-companions discovered a new activity or treatment that worked well, they highlighted it so the rest of us could follow suit. Doris II, for example, applied petroleum jelly to the dried-out and paper-thin skin on my mother's face, as she had done for many years while working full-time in a nursing home. When she noted that my mother's skin tone had improved, other caregiver-companions soon did the same thing.

We also highlighted concerns about Doris that we wanted other caregiver-companions to monitor or take action on, such as getting her to drink more fluids if she had a bladder infection , or getting the physiotherapist to put more air in her wheelchair-seat cushion. For convenience, at the front of the book, we recorded information that we needed as a quick reference, such as phone numbers, the dates when we changed her hearing aid batteries, and my mother's weight.

Thankfully, the information wasn't all clinical. We logged funny and interesting stories to show Doris' wit could momentarily resurface. For example, after Mom had not spoken for days, Joan told Mom, in a coaxing voice, that her chicken dinner looked good and she should try some. Doris gave her a disgruntled look and boldly retorted, "Then *you* eat it!"

All businesses run into problems from time to time and the same holds true for the business of eldercare. Successful companies have an effective monitoring and proactive problem-solving procedure, and so did Doris Inc.

Spending time with Mom's nursing-home staff gave me tremendous insight into how these facilities are run, and allowed me to monitor the care she received, first-hand. As well, every time I visited my mother I read what had gone on in the previous week in Doris' visitor book. I was very quickly brought up to speed on any medical issues that I needed to discuss with the nursing staff while there.

A few times a week, David called our caregiver-companions while they were working to find out how Mom was, hear of any problems, and to talk to Mom herself. Sadly, as her communications skills deteriorated my brother had to do most of the talking.

Our caregiver-companions were also responsible for calling David or me when they found any issues that negatively affected our mother's health, happiness, or comfort. They took this duty seriously as they were my eyes and ears when I wasn't in the nursing home. I don't think I could have created a better monitoring system. One day Jenny suspected that Doris' diaper hadn't been changed for nine hours on the two previous Saturdays so she marked my mother's diaper with a pen before she left after lunch. When she returned for her scheduled evening shift, she saw her pen mark on Doris' diaper, which proved that it had not been changed. After that incident we nicknamed her the "diaper sleuth."

I spoke to the director of care about this problem and was able to provide the evidence of neglect. In this way our caregiver-companions kept the nursing-home staff on their toes. If my mother was neglected in any way, I quickly found out about it. In this particular instance, a valued daytime registered practical nurse had quit due to back problems. Her newly hired replacement was not supervising the personal support workers well enough, and residents started to be ignored. While the director of care did eventually find a great replacement, I decided to address the personal support worker in question. Without revealing that I knew she was at fault, I calmly said that, "It hurts my heart to see my mother left in her wheelchair all day without a break and in a soiled diaper. When you are working in this unit can you look out for my mother to make sure she gets her badly needed rest and a diaper change?" She responded well, volunteered to help, and the problem never recurred.

Once our three care teams gained experience working together, they operated seamlessly and harmoniously. The nursing staff grew to appreciate how receptive David and I were to their suggestions to improve Mom's care. For example, when she reached late-stage Alzheimer's, she slept in her wheelchair more often and had trouble holding her head up, so we agreed to buy her a tilt-back wheelchair.

The nursing staff also grew to respect and value the role our caregiver-companions played, and how well Mom responded to them. They were especially impressed that they could get her to eat better than anyone else. The members of each of our care teams rolled up their sleeves to do whatever it took to keep Doris as healthy, happy, and comfortable as possible.

It took David and me about a year to turn Doris Inc. into a reality, and our venture worked even better in the four years that followed, as we gained more experience with our caregiving process. As children, Mom taught us that we could do whatever we set our minds to, if we believed in ourselves. She was right, and we applied her valuable lesson to her when she needed us most.

DORIS INC.'S FAMILY-CARE LEADERSHIP & CARE-TEAM OPERATIONS APPROACH TO CAREGIVING

The key steps that family caregivers need to take to duplicate Doris Inc.'s approach to caregiving are listed below in chronological order.

Family-Care Leadership

1. Unify the family voice and establish the family-care leadership and caregiving team.
2. Seek good information and advice from medical and elder-care experts.
3. Set goals that articulate the type of care the family agrees to provide.
4. Define the roles and responsibilities of the care teams.
5. Assemble and manage the efforts of the health-care and caregiver-companion teams.
6. Get to know the team members and how they like to work.
7. Show gratitude for demonstrated initiative and dedication.

Care-Team Operations

8. Use communications tools to ensure a well-coordinated caregiving operation.
9. Adopt monitoring and proactive problem-solving procedures.
10. Collaborate with health-care and caregiver-companion teams.

The first priority for families is to unify their family voice, establish family-care leadership over the care and well-being of their aging loved one, and determine who will be on their family caregiving team. Each family has its own group dynamics and complexities, so some families may never be able to unify their voice. If this happens, hopefully other family members can at least validate the primary caregiver in his or her leadership role.

Every family's caregiving situation is also very different. Some seniors will receive care in their home or in their son's or daughter's home, and may die before needing to live in a retirement residence or a nursing home. However, family-care leadership and care-team operations are needed for any frail senior with chronic and debilitating diseases, regardless of where they reside and the type of care provided.

The 10 steps may appear daunting at first. It is important to remember, however, that while Doris Inc. requires family involvement and won't run on autopilot, once it is up and running, the family caregiving workloads and stress levels will be reduced.

That being said, I don't want anyone to feel discouraged if they are not able to activate all elements of the Doris Inc. model. By tackling even some of the steps as well as you can, when you can, I am certain your caregiving road will be easier to travel, and your parent or spouse will receive better care. The rest of the chapters in this book are devoted to preparing family caregivers for their leadership role.

Doris Inc. succeeded beyond our wildest dreams. Mom was happy, receiving much better care, and we had created a great backup system. I also figured out how to fit my caregiving workload into my already hectic life; however, I still worked too hard at everything I did, and having time for fun was a lower priority in my life. It would take a few more years of caregiving experience for me to learn to appreciate life the way Mom did, and to master the art of finding balance.

TOP TIPS

Adopt Doris Inc.'s Approach to Caregiving

- Doris Inc.'s family-care leadership and care-team operations approach to caregiving offers benefits over the common solo firefighter approach:
  - anticipates and plans for needs of seniors as their health declines;

(Continued)

○ provides proactive and good, attentive care;

○ meets needs of whole person, not just physical needs;

○ provides backup support for family caregivers;

○ gives peace of mind and reduces stress on caregivers; and

○ is more time efficient because there will be fewer fires to fight.

Knowledge Harmonizes Family Caregivers

- Good information and advice from medical and elder-care experts leads to good decisions, strong leadership, and more harmony between family members.

- Knowledgeable caregivers feel more in control and are less stressed out.

Lead by Example

- Your health-care team will go the extra mile in caring for your loved one if you:

  ○ speak with one unified family voice;

  ○ demonstrate knowledgeable, dedicated, and passionate leadership over their care; and

  ○ express praise and gratitude when care providers demonstrate initiative and compassion toward your loved one.

Share the Load

- Family members can help, even if they live in another city.

- Caregiver-companions will boost your loved one's sense of self-worth, and give you peace of mind and a lighter workload.

A Caregivers' Daily Logbook Helps Ensure Well-Coordinated Care

- When there is more than one person caring for a sick elder, a caregivers' daily logbook can provide continuity of care:
  - caregivers record the status of a senior's health, their comfort level, food and fluid intake, and any new problems.
  - the next caregiver reads logbook when they first arrive to do a shift, and then carry on where others left off.

Smell the Roses

- Take time to enjoy and appreciate special moments with your aging mom, dad, or spouse, and love them with all your heart. If you do, you will have no regrets and more wonderful memories.

$$\textbf{\large{3}}$$

Finding Balance in My Life

For most of the years that I cared for my mother I was running my own marketing consulting practice, which had an unpredictable workload. I was either overwhelmed with too much work and not enough time to complete it, or I had a brief lull to write proposals for new projects. My personal life often took a backseat. I seemed to always be in a hurry with little or no time for fun and relaxation—the definition of unbalanced. And I was not alone.

According to Statistics Canada, 2.7 million Canadians in the population aged 45 and older provided some form of unpaid care to seniors with long-term health problems in 2007.[1] That was one in five people in that 45+ age group. Adults like me, who were between the ages of 45 and 64, provided three-quarters of the eldercare. Seniors caring for a spouse provided the balance of care.

The tasks that caregivers performed were jobs inside and outside a senior's house; providing transportation and personal care; and looking after, care management that involved scheduling or coordinating tasks, such as hiring, monitoring, and dismissing professional help, managing finances, making appointments, and negotiating provision of services. Many caregivers reported having multiple responsibilities. In 2007, more than half of them

---

[1] Statistics Canada, *Canadian Social Trends*, "Eldercare: What we know today," p 48–56, reporting on the General Social Survey, 2007, Catalogue no. 11-008.

were working at a paid job at the time, and because 43 per cent of caregivers were between the ages of 45 and 54 they likely still had children living at home.

In the cycle of life, there is a time to be born, to love, to give birth, to parent, to reap the rewards of having a spouse and children, to have fun, to be a caregiver for a parent and later for a spouse, to mourn, and a time to receive caregiving when our final years, months, and days draw near. While caregiving for a loved one is a considerable responsibility, there is a season when we should return our parent's and spouse's love in this unselfish manner.

I believe that it was my time to step up to the plate and seize my caregiving role with generosity and grace; however, I also felt that I needed courage and wisdom to find a state of equilibrium where my mother's needs and mine were both being met. Primary caregivers need backup not just to cover for sickness and time off, but also to ensure that the end goal is met: that their loved one is properly cared for. Caregiving is too big a job for one person. Primary caregivers also need to learn to pace themselves. In the 2007 Statistics Canada General Social Survey, caregivers aged 45 to 64 had already been providing care for five years, and those 65 and older had been providing care for seven years.

My caregiving role lasted for seven years, and Mom certainly had her share of medical emergencies during that time. After a year and a half of caregiving, David and I set up Doris Inc.; however, it would take me another two years to learn how to have a happy, healthy, and rewarding life while caregiving. I accomplished this feat by doing five things: finding the right type of support; building coping skills; managing stress; making compromises and setting limits; and redefining life balance.

FIND THE RIGHT TYPE OF SUPPORT

Caregivers, who are often too reluctant or too stubborn to ask for help, could learn from my mother's ability to request assistance from people with the greatest of ease. She was tenacious in a charming sweet way. Her motto was, "There's no harm in asking. You will be amazed by what wishes will be granted."

When Doris was in her 70s, she and her good friend Julie used to walk a half-mile to a park in Cobourg overlooking Lake Ontario, and back home again. Mom thought that it would be great to have a bench there so they could rest awhile before starting home. She wrote a letter to her town councillor requesting that a bench be placed in the park. To everyone's surprise, within two months the town granted Mom her wish and placed a wooden bench in the park, proving that there is indeed no harm in asking.

Finding balance in life and asking for help go hand in hand. Asking for the right type of support from resources that are readily available will greatly improve a caregiver's chance at finding both. The four types of support that caregivers will likely need are: informational, care and financial management, emotional, and task- and care-oriented.

Four Types of Support Needed

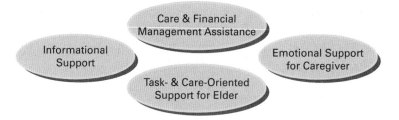

Informational Support

Quick access to reliable information is crucial for a caregiver not only to perform his or her duties well but also to feel in control.

Types of Support	Available Resources
Informational	
• Advice and suggestions • Contacts and referrals for support services • Government-funded services and subsidies • Information about diseases that affect seniors	• Family doctor, geriatrician • Hospital discharge planner and provincial community care agency • Health charities

There are many informational resources available, such as provincial community care agencies and health charities, that provide relevant information, answer questions, offer advice, and make referrals. They often have chapters in each province, so caregivers can get support for their loved one in their community.

The provincial community care agency assigns your family a case manager, who will assess your loved one's needs while they are living at home or while they are in the hospital before they are discharged. The case manager coordinates the delivery of government-funded home care that they feel is necessary, such as a nurse, personal support workers, lab services, physiotherapist, occupational therapist, speech therapist, social worker, respite for a caregiver, nutritional counselling, and medical supplies and equipment. She or he may also recommend community support services that families can access at their own cost. Importantly, the provincial community care agencies are also the single point of entry to nursing homes. They handle the clinical assessment to determine if a senior qualifies to be in a nursing home, as well as the application process.

In Ontario, the Community Care Access Centre (CCAC) referred me to cleaning ladies, who worked for seniors at a reasonable price, and to local meal-preparation services. The CCAC also organized home care for my mother after she suffered serious complications from surgery to insert a pacemaker. Care included regular visits from a registered nurse to change her dressings and check her vital signs. A personal support worker came each day for a few hours to bathe and dress her, as well as cook a light meal until Mom was strong enough to do so on her own. Later, the agency guided me through the nursing-home placement process.

Health charities provide extensive educational support to help families better understand how a disease will progress over time and the care that will be required. They also offer reliable and up-to-date information on a broad range of topics, often including the names of medical specialists and clinics. The Alzheimer Society of Canada, for example, answered many of our questions concerning the stages of the disease, how to get Mom to eat, where to find a dementia-friendly dentist, and how to communicate with her in the disease's final stage.

A wealth of information can also be found on the federal government website, Seniors Canada Online (www.seniors.gc.ca), which links to various programs and services.

Care and Financial Management Assistance

You may need assistance from an eldercare consultant to manage the care of your loved one, because hiring, scheduling, and monitoring care are ongoing and time-consuming duties. Managing an elder's financial affairs is another area that can usually benefit from the aid of accredited financial specialists, such as accountants and investment advisors.

Types of Support	Available Resources
Care Management	
• Scheduling and coordinating caregiving tasks • Hiring, monitoring, and dismissing professional help • Negotiating provision of services	• Shared responsibilities with family members • Eldercare consultant
Financial Management	
• Paying bills • Managing bank accounts and investments • Completing income tax return	• Family member, bank, trust company • Family expert, investment advisor, trust company • Family expert, accountant

Emotional Support

Emotional support is vital to caregivers' physical and mental health and sanity, because while they are consumed by their day-to-day tasks, they are watching their loved one decline and slowly die. Fortunately, there are excellent free resources available. Health charities offer caregiver support groups as well as counselling for people living with a disease and for their family. While I was on the board of directors of Parkinson Society Canada, a fellow board member confessed to me one day that the counselling he received saved his life. He had become so depressed by his diagnosis of Parkinson's disease, at the age of 47, that he considered suicide. With the society's support, he no longer defines himself by his disease and has become one of the charity's strongest advocates in the fight to find a cure for this debilitating neurological disease.

Backup respite support is also essential. Adult daycare, provincial community care agencies' home-care programs, short stays in a nursing home or retirement residence, home-support service companies and volunteers are available.

Types of Support	Available Resources
Emotional	
• Confidant or sounding board • Family counselling • Caregiver support group	• Sibling, spouse, or friend • Hospital discharge planners • Health charities
Respite	
• Backup for primary caregivers so they can have a life of their own • Ongoing companionship and comfort care for senior • A day, a weekend, a week or two, or a month stay for senior	• Family, friends, and neighbours • Home-support service companies • Caregiver-companions hired privately or through an agency • Pastoral care • Adult day-care services and seniors' centres • Provincial community care agencies • Short stays in nursing homes or retirement residences

Task- and Care-Oriented Support

Primary caregivers will also need to find extensive support for their ailing senior to handle household chores, escorted transportation to medical appointments, arrange a medical alert system if they live alone, administer professional health and personal care, and supply specialized assistive devices, such as walkers, wheelchairs, and hearing aids. This type of support reduces the workload of caregivers, allowing them to focus on managing the care process, which is an important part of their leadership role.

Types of Support	Available Resources
Household Chores	
• House cleaning, maintenance, and repairs • Meal preparation and laundry • Lawn cutting and snow shovelling • Shopping	• Family, friends, and neighbours • Community support service agencies on a volunteer or small-fee basis • Individuals or company services for hire
Transportation	
• Transit for shopping, appointments, and social activities when senior can no longer drive, but still lives independently • Escorted transit to medical appointments when senior no longer lives independently	• Family, friends, and neighbours • Community volunteers • Pastoral care and volunteers from local churches • Taxi services • Wheelchair-accessible bus service • Emergency and non-emergency ambulances
Medical Alert System	
• Regular checks by phone or in person for senior who lives alone • Personal emergency-response system with a two-way voice communicator and personal help button	• Family, friends, neighbours, and volunteers • Commercial service providers

(Continued)

Types of Support	Available Resources
Medical & Personal Care	
• Ongoing health care • Home care, such as nursing and personal care, occupational and physiotherapy • Acute care • Supportive and assisted living • 24-hour nursing and personal care • Hospice palliative care	• Family doctor and/or geriatrician • Provincial community-care agencies • Nursing-home care agencies • Hospital • Retirement residences and seniors' housing • Nursing home • Nursing home, hospital palliative-care unit, and hospice organization volunteers
Assistive Devices	
• Mobility aids, such as walkers and wheelchairs, and specialized products, such as hearing aids, oxygen, and artificial limbs	• Provincial community care agencies • Home health-care pharmacies

Family members can be one of the most reliable resources because they have an emotional attachment to the ailing senior. Even if siblings live in a different city they can play a vital role in care and financial management. It's an electronic world. All they need is a phone, computer, e-mail, and the Internet.

A caregiver's spouse and children can also help by relieving them of household chores at home, and becoming a sounding board for them to vent their worries and frustrations. Friends and neighbours can also lend a hand by helping with chores, transportation, and companionship. Primary caregivers just need to ask, and then delegate specific duties, keeping in mind the type of help required, and the talents and availability of each family, friend, or neighbour volunteer.

BUILD COPING SKILLS

Even with the right type of support, caring for an aging parent can become both physically and emotionally exhausting if their illness becomes very complex, incapacitating, or lasts a long time.

As Mom would say, "When life throws you a curve, it's to teach you how to bend." Facing adversity in life teaches us how to be flexible, but it's easy to get so entrenched in caregiving and not recognize the increasing demands that we ignore gradual changes in our own health, such as rising blood pressure. When this happens we can lose sight of the toll that is being taken on us.

Developing coping skills increases our physical, mental, and emotional capacities to handle the caregiving role. Drawing upon my business and caregiving experiences I developed four coping skills: prepare for emergencies, improve time-management skills, make yourself a priority, and develop your spirituality.

Prepare for Emergencies

I prepared a contact list of Mom's health-care specialists, a list of her medications for the hospital, and a backup plan if I got sick or was away when an emergency occurred. That way I minimized the stress that always comes with the need for urgent care.

Improve Time-Management Skills

I needed to accomplish more each day than I did before I became a caregiver, so I re-adjusted my priorities whenever my plate became too full. Then, with the help of a weekly to-do list, I focused on accomplishing my top priorities. I also eliminated time wasters, by learning to say no to unreasonable requests and I adopted time savers, such as shopping in non-peak periods and on-line, and paying bills while waiting in doctor's offices.

Make Yourself a Priority

I made myself a priority, so that my own health didn't decline. This meant sleeping six to eight hours each night, eating balanced and nutritious meals, drinking six to eight glasses of water a day, exercising 30 to 60 minutes six days a week, keeping my medical appointments, and taking time off from caregiving.

Develop Your Spirituality

As I've mentioned, caregiving can be all-encompassing and you can easily lose perspective and feel as if you are all alone. Developing your spirituality can help. Adopting a positive attitude by counting my many blessings in life helped me. I also prayed for guidance, especially when David and I had tough decisions to make. Of course, each one of us has our own spiritual path; taking the time to meditate on bigger questions and gaining peace of mind is an important part of coping.

For a more complete list of coping skills, see page 56–58.

MANAGE STRESS

Stress comes with the territory of caregiving as adult children support their parents through unsettling life-changing transitions, such as losing a spouse, losing health, and losing independence. Managing stress, therefore, is critical.

Everyone experiences stress differently, some with more tolerance than others. That is why each of us must recognize the emotional and physical warning signs of too much stress. The Alzheimer Society of Canada lists the warning signs as follows:

Emotional Signs of Stress	Physical Signs of Stress
Sleeplessness	Upset stomach
Irritability	Back pain
Depression	Muscle tension
Lack of concentration	Headaches or other pain
Emotional volatility	Racing heartbeat
Anger	Shortness of breath
Anxiety	Dizziness or faintness
Negative thinking	Shaking
Increased forgetfulness	Sweating

The triggers that cause people to feel stress vary from person to person, so it's important to learn what our stress triggers are and thus find a more positive response than experiencing stress. For me, it's a messy house, especially when I am expecting visitors, so while caring for Mom, I hired someone to clean our house every two weeks. Worry is another of my stress triggers; I used to fret over each new health problem that Mom developed. By learning as much as I could about her medical conditions, and how they would affect her over time, I felt more in control of the situation. This helped me to make better and proactive decisions so I worried less about her.

In my caregiving journey, I learned how to diffuse my feelings of stress. Here is a list of the stress busters that have worked for me and other caregivers:

- Don't bottle up your feelings. Find a sounding board, such as a friend or spouse, to vent your worries and frustrations.
- Take deep breaths, for a few minutes at a time, when totally stressed out.
- Exercise to reduce tension—even a brisk walk can help.
- Take regular mini-breaks from caregiving.

In my life, and especially in my caregiving role, I have found stress relief, comfort, and guidance from the theologian Reinhold Niebuhr's "The Serenity Prayer," which has been adopted by Alcoholics Anonymous:

The Serenity Prayer

God, grant me the serenity
To accept the things I cannot change;
Courage to change the things I can;
And the wisdom to know the difference.

This prayer gave me the guidance to encourage Mom's doctor to prescribe a medication to slow the progression of Alzheimer's disease, but to accept the reality that I couldn't stop or reverse the course of the illness that was destroying her brain. Instead, I channelled my energy into fighting this insidious disease. I did this by mentally stimulating my mother: reading to her, and involving her in conversations and activities. I also encouraged her to function as well as she could, using her remaining capabilities, especially her five senses.

Realistically, caregivers are likely to find themselves in crisis mode from time to time as they cope with medical emergencies; however, if a crisis mode becomes the norm, the unrelenting stress will be harmful to everyone. It is easy to see how caregiver burnout can happen as we get so caught up in the emotional roller coaster of caring for our parent or spouse. At first, we are in denial about the seriousness of their illness. Next, we become hopeful that their health will improve. Eventually, we underestimate the amount of help they will need from us and others. Once our loved one moves into a nursing home, we fear that health-care professionals will neglect our parent or spouse, or won't understand their special needs as well as we do. When this happens, we try to compensate by devoting even more time to caring for our loved one.

We can become selfless, lowering the priority on our own needs, and convince ourselves that we can manage on fewer hours of sleep, rushed meals, and a limited social life. There is also a natural tendency to feel guilty every time we tend to our own needs; however, we must control our emotions and our life, and remember that we don't need to be a hero. Our loved one wouldn't want us to sacrifice our health to care for them. Most importantly, we must remember that if we get sick, we can't take care of our loved one.

Over time, stress can lead to high blood pressure and a weakened immune system, which can decrease the body's ability to fight infections and diseases, and avoid accidents. The telltale warning signs of caregiver burnout include the following:

- sleeplessness or exhaustion
- new medical problems
- weight loss or gain
- depression, anxiety, irritability, or anger
- impatience and resentment toward the senior and/or other family members

- feeling helpless, or hopeless, and overwhelmed most of the time
- neglect of personal care and other aspects of a person's life
- excesses of food, medications, smoking, alcohol, or caffeine
- refusal to get help or take a break
- social withdrawal

MAKING COMPROMISES AND SETTING LIMITS

Balancing our caregiving responsibilities with other demands on our time requires us to make compromises and set limits on the care we are willing and able to provide. Once that is sorted out, we must find others to meet the care needs of our parent or spouse that we aren't able to handle.

Caregivers need to be honest with themselves, assess their current obligations and abilities, and what they are realistically able to handle. If their health is failing too, if they live in another city, or have a demanding full-time job, they will require more external help than other caregivers.

Without setting limits, caregiving duties will gradually start to run their life as their loved one's health declines. When this happens the rest of their life will be neglected, and an emotional vicious circle may unfold. They may resent their loved one, they may exhibit their anger and impatience, and then feel guilty that they resent them, and didn't treat them as well as they should have.

Every caregiver is very different and needs to determine their own definition of balance that takes into account the elements of their life that are most important to them. As well, they should consider their values, energy level, work ethic, and personal needs, such as having an active social life or pursuing a career.

Some very nurturing primary caregivers who have strong family values willingly give up their careers, and much of their free time, to provide eldercare in their home for a period of time. For them, their life is more fulfilling that way, and they would be out of balance if they tried to maintain a demanding career at the same time.

For others, like me, having a career is an important part of their lives, so they need more help to care for their loved one, in order to still have a rewarding life. For still other caregivers, working full time is a financial necessity, as is having their chronically ill parent or spouse live with them. Finding balance is more difficult under these circumstances but it is possible by organizing a volunteer care team, building coping skills, managing their stress level, and making some compromises.

Early on I set one limit on my caregiving duties. I decided to not move my mother to a Toronto nursing home from Cobourg, where she had lived for 30 years. I knew that if I did, I would have felt enormous self-inflicted pressure to visit her every day, because she would have become even more dependent upon me. She would not have had any friends, neighbours, or pastoral care visitors, and rightly or wrongly, I didn't think big-city support would be as compassionate and personal as that in a small town.

After a few years' of caregiving, I made several compromises to regain balance in my life that worked very well. Professionally, I reduced the number of clients that I handled at one time; I cut my workweek from six to four days a week. This allowed me to fit my care-management duties into a half-day during business hours, when I needed to make calls; and my household chores into the rest of that day, leaving me the weekends to spend with my family.

I made other compromises, too. For the first three years of caregiving, I declined volunteer responsibilities—Mom was all the "volunteer" work I could handle. I also didn't see my friends as much; instead, we kept in touch via e-mail. I also became friends with the caregiver-companions that I had hired at that point.

What I did not compromise, however, was my loving relationship with my mother. And yet, I remember one dark moment early on in my caregiving role when I let my caregiving duties consume me. I became so concerned about Mom not eating well enough and losing weight that I became quite bossy during one particular lunch hour in the hospital dining room. I tried to force her to eat, but to my shocking surprise she uncharacteristically hurled food at me.

On the rare occasion that I witnessed my mother's wrath, it had never been directed at me. Horrified and ashamed of myself, I took Doris back to her room, and brought some apple-sauce, cranberry juice, and chocolate-chip cookies with us. About an hour later, I asked Mom if she was hungry enough to eat her dessert. She confessed that she was and ate her dessert without any assistance from me. Since that fateful day, I was slower and gentler with her and devoted more time to nurturing our friendship.

REDEFINE LIFE BALANCE

Looking back over the past seven years, I realize that caregiving is an opportunity for personal growth, which is an important life endeavour. As my mother's priest, Canon Peter Walker, put it, "Growth is the only evidence of life, and if you aren't growing you are declining." The experience gave me strength, confidence, and a real sense of accomplishment. I am better prepared for adversity when it next strikes.

I also take better care of myself and live much more in the present, than the past, and try to worry less about the future. This is a lesson that I learned from my mother, who, with the progression of Alzheimer's, could no longer remember the past, or comprehend the future.

We shared treasured moments in the present using sight, smell, hearing, and touch. We experienced the wind in our face, the warmth of the sun, the scent and beauty of flowers, and the boisterous excitement of two squawking seagulls fighting over a hamburger bun.

My priorities and values have changed so much since becoming a caregiver, that the common way of thinking about work-life balance now seems too simplistic to capture all that matters in life.

Instead, I think our goal should be to have a happy, healthy, and rewarding life while caregiving—and after. A deeper sense of contentment is achievable with a rewarding life-balance equation that resembles a house with three doors and a foundation:

Rewarding Life-Balance Equation

We need a solid foundation of self-care to have the energy and endurance to get the most out of life. With this in place, there are three doors to our life activities that we can choose to open in our remaining waking hours: paid work and chores; enjoying life with family, friends, neighbours, and ourselves; and altruism. Finding a good balance between the three life activities is the secret to having a rewarding life.

Life Activities	Examples	Rewards
Paid Work and Chores	• Career, employment • Household and personal tasks	• Money, security, success • Comfort • Sense of accomplishment
Enjoying Life	• Social life with spouse, family, and friends • Leisure and entertainment activities	• Love • Sense of belonging • Fun and pleasure
Altruism	• Caregiving and helping others in need • Acts of kindness and generosity • Volunteerism • Donations	• Joy • Purpose in life • Sense of accomplishment • Satisfaction in giving back

TOP TIPS

Finding Life Balance and Asking for Help Go Hand in Hand

- Ask for the right type of support from resources that are readily available to improve your chance of success in finding both help and life balance.
- Draw upon four types of support: informational, care and financial management, emotional, and task- and care-oriented.

Knowledge is Power So Research and Learn

- Gain reliable information, referrals, and advice to feel in control over your caregiving duties.

Build Coping Skills

- Prepare for emergencies, improve your time-management skills, make yourself a priority, and develop your spirituality.

Manage Stress

- Recognize your own physical and emotional warning signs of stress.
- Recognize and avoid your stress triggers, such as excessive worrying.
- Adopt stress busters, such as finding a sounding board to vent frustrations.

Make Compromises and Set Limits

- Determine what you will and will not give up to take on your caregiving duties.
- Find others to meet the care needs of your loved one that you won't be able to handle.

(Continued)

Build a Strong Self-Care Foundation

- To take care of someone else, you have to take care of yourself.

Stomp Out Caregiver Burnout

- Regain control of your caregiving life by:
  - taking a break from caregiving to gain perspective;
  - setting limits and saying no to unreasonable requests;
  - finding supporters to share your caregiving work-load; and
  - rebuilding your self-care foundation.

COPING SKILLS FOR CAREGIVERS

Prepare for Emergencies

- Develop a list of important people and their contact information, including your loved one's family doctor and other health-care specialists.
- Prepare a list of the senior's medications that can accompany them to the hospital.
- Develop a backup plan if you get sick or aren't available, or if hired help doesn't show up.

Improve Time-Management Skills

- Readjust priorities when your plate is too full.

- Stay focused on top priorities with the help of a weekly to-do list.
- Eliminate time wasters by saying no to unreasonable requests.
- Adopt time savers, such as shopping in non-peak periods or on-line.
- Multi-task, by paying bills while waiting for medical appointments, for example.
- Break down large tasks, such as moving a parent, into smaller steps, and tackle them one at a time.
- Use e-mails to handle care coordination and follow-up responsibilities.

Make Yourself a Priority

- Don't cancel your medical appointments.
- Make time for your own personal care.
- Don't give up your vacations and take regular mini-breaks from caregiving.
- Boost your stamina with nutritious foods, proper hydration, regular exercise, and enough sleep.
- Put yourself on pause an hour before going to bed so you will get a good night's sleep. During that time do whatever will calm your mind and body, such as taking a hot bath, reading a book, watching TV, or listening to soothing music.
- Find opportunities to laugh and have fun.
- Stay connected with friends, even if it is by e-mail, Facebook, or by inviting them over while you are caregiving.

(Continued)

Develop Your Spirituality

- Adopt peaceful spiritual rituals:
  - Meditate.
  - Pray to a higher power so you remember that you are not alone or abandoned, even though it may feel that way.
  - Count your blessings to help develop a positive attitude and to put your caregiving role into perspective.
  - Use relaxing visualization techniques, such as picturing a beautiful lake.
  - Spend peaceful time relaxing with nature.

$$\textbf{(4)}$$

Planning for the Stages
of Decline

In February 1999, Mom endured a life-threatening medical crisis. She was preparing dinner one evening when suddenly she fell to the floor and passed out, her face hitting the floor with a heavy thud. Dad was working in the basement when he heard the pans crashing and came running up the stairs to the kitchen.

While he looked at my mother helplessly, not quite sure what he should do, she came to. Her forehead and eye were bruised and her arms and legs were scraped and bleeding. Dad took Mom to the hospital where the emergency room employees looked at him suspiciously, suspecting that he might have caused her injuries.

My mother was diagnosed with cardiac arrhythmia, which meant her heart wasn't beating fast enough at times to pump enough blood for her body. When her brain didn't receive enough blood, she became light-headed and fainted. The solution was simple: the surgeon would insert a pacemaker to monitor her heart. When her heart beat fewer than 60 times a minute, the pacemaker would stimulate the heart ventricle with a short low voltage pulse, causing it to beat faster, and maintain the proper blood supply.

Doris was sent by ambulance to the Peterborough regional hospital for the surgery with only a day's notice, so neither Dad nor I accompanied Mom. Her sister had had the same operation a few years earlier without any complications, so we thought it would be a routine procedure. Besides, I was bogged down with consulting-project deadlines so I planned to visit my mother the next morning, on Saturday, when she was expected to be back in the Cobourg hospital.

It was a bitter cold Friday evening when my phone rang in Toronto, interrupting my worried thoughts about my mother's operation. It was the surgeon: "Your mother is in the intensive care unit, with a punctured lung, and I don't know if she will pull through. I feel very bad. This has never happened to me before."

I told him that we would be at the Peterborough hospital in the morning. Instantly childhood memories of my mother and me flooded my mind. I was furious with myself for not taking the day off work to accompany her on what could have been her last day alive.

Mitch and I picked up my father then drove to the hospital. We anxiously entered the ICU to the unmistakable sound of my mother, quite high on drugs, throwing out witty one-liners and laughing exuberantly with the nurses. It was such a wonderful sound!

Her recovery took eight months and required home visits from health-care professionals, including a nurse and personal support workers to bathe her and cook light meals. Fortunately, no drastic lifestyle or living arrangement changes were necessary. However, Mom became frail while convalescing and required more support from neighbours, friends, a cleaning lady, and David and me, so that she and Dad could remain in their home.

In hindsight, I realized that David and I were completely unprepared to support our parents through their inevitable decline. We didn't understand what their increasing care needs would be, what living arrangement options existed, and if these options were available in the Cobourg area. As well, we didn't know our parents' end-of-life wishes. In fact, what we *didn't* know far exceeded what we *did*, and the little we *did* know wasn't good;

our parents had not made any funeral arrangements yet, despite their advanced ages.

Most of us like to plan for the future: vacations, Christmases with our family, a new home, or our retirement. However, we tend to avoid thinking about or planning for the future care needs of our aging parents and ourselves until a crisis jolts us into action. David and I were no exceptions. As our nation's population ages, however, eldercare will become as common and necessary as childcare.

Without knowledge and planning, any elder crisis may become worse when family caregivers are suddenly forced to educate themselves and make hasty decisions. When this happens, aging loved ones are less likely to receive well-orchestrated care, or have input into their well-being.

Developing an *advance care plan* while seniors are still healthy and able to communicate their wishes will help ensure that they will live as independently as they can for as long as they can, receive the right level of care at all stages of their decline, avoid preventable accidents, and make their end-of-life wishes known. The key elements of an advance care plan should be to plan for increasing care needs and changes in living arrangements, prepare advance care directives, make funeral arrangements, and establish a family-care leadership and caregiving team in waiting.

PLAN FOR INCREASING CARE NEEDS

Mom's slide from living independently with Dad, receiving help only with some household chores, to dependent living in a nursing home took only five years. During this time, I learned that seniors may go through natural stages of physical and/or mental decline that affect their ability to perform tasks of daily living. While not everyone will go through all four stages of decline, and the length of time spent at each stage will vary greatly, the need for increasing care in a loved one's final years of life can reasonably be expected. With this knowledge, families can map out their caregiving journey that most likely lies ahead.

Probable Stages of Elder Decline

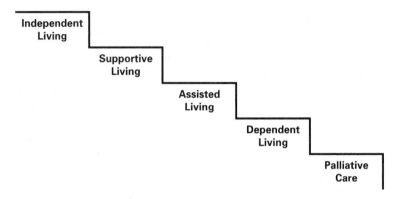

Independent Living

Seniors who have the mental and physical ability to live independently and determine their own destiny, as they did when they were younger, don't need much help from their family. They may be showing early signs of aging, such as greying hair and wrinkles, but they can usually manage their household chores on their own. They may even be caring for their own parents.

Supportive-Living Stage

With advancing age, seniors typically step onto the ladder of decline. Their joints become stiffer, they lose bone and muscle mass, and stamina. As well, eyesight and hearing often diminish, and chronic diseases, such as diabetes, heart disease, and arthritis may start to raise their ugly heads.

At this point, seniors need a watchful eye from their children and neighbours, because it is usually the small changes, such as difficulty with household chores, cooking, taking medications, or driving that indicate that they are transitioning into the supportive-living stage. Over time, some seniors will start to neglect their personal appearance and have memory and behavioural problems. When my parents were in their late 70s,

I saw a number of warning signs that they needed support to continue living in their own home. The house wasn't as clean, mail and bills were piled up in their spare bedroom, and the fridge contained spoiled food. The exterior of the house, garden, and lawn weren't as well kept as they used to be, and my parents' personal appearance was starting to look dowdy. As well, my father became a nervous driver and would only drive his prized white Oldsmobile Cutlass Ciera as far as the local grocery store.

Warning Signs that Seniors Have Reached the Supportive-Living Stage

Area of Neglect	Warning Signs
Personal Appearance	• Poor hygiene, hair untidy or greasy • Dressing poorly or inappropriately • Bruises and other signs of trauma, falls, or abuse
Housekeeping	• Dirty and cluttered house, and laundry piling up • House maintenance and repairs neglected inside and out • Gardens and lawn neglected • Snow not being shovelled
Eating	• Significant or unexplained weight loss or gain • Problems preparing food • Fridge in disarray or empty, food with long past expiry dates or spoiled
Medication Mix-ups	• Medications expired, unfilled, or not being taken • Confusion about when and why medications should be taken
Memory Problems	• Leaving stove or lights on • Unopened or unpaid bills • Forgotten appointments • Calling repeatedly or forgetting to call
Behavioural Problems	• Spending money inappropriately • Reclusive, anti-social behaviour, sadness or anxiety • Fewer invitations to the home • Driving unsafely, having accidents

At this juncture, family members need to get involved and support their loved ones, so they can live as independently as they can for as long as they can. They must do so, however, with great diplomacy and respect, because their parents or spouse are adults and have the legal right to make their own decisions, as long as they are deemed mentally capable. They may need information about their options, but ultimately it is their choice how they live.

Often during this stage, a married senior loses his or her spouse. This is a life-changing event. Up to this point, each spouse typically performed the household tasks that they could still do, and their combined efforts allowed them to live on their own, in a co-dependent state, with just a little help. Losing a spouse means that many tasks won't get done, and the probability that the surviving spouse can live on their own is greatly reduced. Since men tend to marry women younger than themselves and women have a longer life expectancy, it is more likely that wives and mothers will be left alone in their final years.

Assisted-Living Stage

The risk that seniors will have a medical emergency, such as a bad fall or a stroke, increases on this steadfast stepladder of decline. It may be a temporary setback, but most often it is the beginning of a more rapid decline in health. This is what happened with my mother; she broke her leg and never walked again, and soon her dementia symptoms became much worse.

With increasing inactivity and frailty, seniors decline to the assisted-living stage. They usually can no longer drive, cook their own meals, or take care of their home, and they may require help bathing, dressing, getting up from chairs, and walking. By this time, they often have cognitive or multiple health problems, which make them vulnerable to further medical mishaps. The table below lists the recognizable warning signs that it may be unsafe for your loved one to live alone, and a change in living arrangements should be considered.

Warning Signs that Elders Have Reached the Assisted-Living Stage

Area of Decline	Warning Signs
Physical Limitations	• Difficulty walking, climbing stairs, or rising from a chair • Losing balance, and at high risk of falling • Diminished eyesight and hearing
Behavioural Problems	• Lack of initiative and social withdrawal • Memory loss affecting daily activities • Inability to plan their activities
Health Problems	• Chronic and more complex debilitating illnesses requiring medical supervision

Even when seniors reach the assisted-living stage, they often fail to anticipate and plan for the possibility that they may eventually need to live in a nursing home. While loved ones are still relatively well but starting to decline, families should help them make some choices about which nursing homes they like best, just in case they need one. That way, if they have a medical emergency and become a high priority for a nursing-home placement, they will have the advantage of getting on the waiting list for their preferred facilities.

Dependent-Living Stage

When a loved one's ability to perform activities of daily living declines considerably or their illnesses grow very complex, they become totally dependent on their family and health-care professionals for their well-being. Some may reach this stage only in the last few weeks of their life in an acute-care hospital, after suffering a stroke or congestive heart failure, for example. However, elders with chronic debilitating diseases, such as dementia, may remain in the totally dependent-living stage for many years. In that case, they may need to live in a nursing home or with family members, augmented by nursing and personal care.

Geriatricians have a grading system for evaluating each patient's life situation and their self-care needs. They assess a senior's ability to perform, unassisted, the basic activities of daily life (ADLs) of eating, dressing, bathing, using the toilet, and moving from a bed to a chair and to the toilet. This assessment helps health-care professionals determine when an elder has reached the dependent-living stage, and qualifies to be admitted to a nursing home. Family members should complete their own ongoing assessment, so they can determine when their parent or spouse needs much more attentive round-the-clock nursing and personal care.

Since there are long waiting lists in some regions of Canada for nursing-home placements, it is important for people to get on the waiting list for their preferred long-term care home as soon as they qualify for admission. If families want to and can afford to hire professional nursing care in their home, then applying for a nursing-home placement may be unnecessary.

Palliative-Care Stage

When your loved one becomes seriously ill and no medical intervention can reverse his or her decline, hospice palliative care will make them more comfortable and manage the pain in their last months, weeks, or days of life.

PLAN FOR CHANGES TO LIVING ARRANGEMENTS

Adult children are often reluctant to have a conversation with their aging parents about their death and care needs as their health declines, and the possibility of having to leave their beloved home. Sons and daughters find themselves in an awkward and intimidating role of parenting their parents. Likewise, seniors avoid the subject for fear of losing their independence or being abandoned by their family if they end up in a nursing home. Ironically, they will have more control, if they express their lifestyle and living arrangement preferences and end-of-life wishes to their family before their health declines.

Ideally, conversations about future care plans and the possible changes to living arrangements should occur when an aging loved one is in their 70s or younger and still healthy and able to discuss this issue objectively. The topic may be easier to address at that time because their decline will be perceived as a long way off. Family members should be frank about whether or not they want to care for their loved one in their own home. Even if a son or daughter wishes to do so for a number of years, they may realistically need to clarify to their parents that a nursing home may be the best option, if they reach the dependent-living stage. The cost of hiring nursing and round-the-clock personal care in a home may be prohibitive, and take too great a toll on their family.

If adult children feel they will be unable to care for their parent or parents in their own home, they should raise the questions of what other living arrangements exist, and which ones the parents or spouse prefer. Research will help everyone make informed decisions.

Candidly discuss the pros and cons of various options for both caregivers and care receivers. That way seniors may be less likely to develop unrealistic expectations, and try to convince a son or daughter to promise to never put them in a nursing home.

PREPARE ADVANCE CARE DIRECTIVES

Making choices about our own personal and medical care is a human right that can be lost if we lose consciousness, are in a coma, or are unable to understand the consequences of making or not making a decision. This can happen if we have an illness, such as a stroke or dementia, or an accident.

Advance care directives give someone whom we trust the information and authority to act on our wishes, when making decisions about medical treatment, food, housing, clothing, hygiene, and safety. Legally appointing a substitute decision-maker and communicating our wishes are the two components of advance care directives that all adults should put in place, while they are healthy and mentally capable.

Appoint a Substitute Decision-Maker

A Power of Attorney for Personal Care is the legal document in Ontario that gives us the ability to choose who we want to be our substitute decision-maker, and act on our behalf regarding the type of care we want. While the term may be different, all provinces have regulations that give citizens the right to appoint a substitute decision-maker. This individual, also called an attorney, can only use his or her power if we have been deemed to be mentally incapable of making our own medical-treatment decisions.

When my parents were in their late 70s, they had a lawyer help them prepare their wills. The lawyer recommended that they also put in place Power of Attorney for Personal Care documents at that time, while they were both mentally competent. They appointed David and me, jointly and severally, their attorneys in 1995, which meant we could act in concert, or individually.

This proved to be a very wise decision because seven years later Dad lost consciousness three days before he died of congestive heart failure. Mom and I were encouraged by nursing staff to sign a do-not-resuscitate order for Dad when his kidneys started to shut down. We decided to do so only after consulting with the attending physician. Two years after that, Mom developed Alzheimer's disease and was deemed mentally incompetent to make her own decisions. David and I used our attorney status frequently to take good care of her in her final years.

A substitute decision-maker should be someone we trust who knows us very well, lives nearby, is compassionate, has high moral standards, is willing and able to make care decisions on our behalf, and can do so decisively after weighing all options. Legally, a substitute decision-maker can't be someone who is paid to provide us with personal care, such as a nurse or doctor. Once we have appointed our attorney or attorneys, it is prudent to keep their contact information in our wallet so they can be reached quickly if we become incapacitated.

Lawyers stress the importance of naming the most appropriate persons to be substitute decision-makers. For example, if a widow has four children it is likely that some would be better candidates than others, and while it would be ludicrous to name all four in an effort to be even-handed, it would be short-sighted to name only one. If the one named becomes incapable of acting, through death or incapacity, or is unavailable when needed, then there would be no backup legally appointed attorney.

If someone becomes incapacitated and has not legally appointed a substitute decision-maker, or their attorney is unable or is unwilling to act, then a stand-in person will be authorized to make health and personal care decisions for the individual. In Ontario, the Health Care Consent Act lists a hierarchy of people who are authorized to become a substitute decision-maker.

1. Representative appointed by the Consent and Capacity Board
2. Spouse or partner
3. Child, if they are at least 16 years of age
4. Parent
5. Brother or sister
6. Other relative
7. Guardian appointed by a court

The highest-ranking person on the list is called on to act first. Family or friends can apply to become a representative of the patient to make health-care decisions. If there is no one on the list willing and able to act, or available to act, then a court-appointed guardian would provide treatment consent, or refusal of consent, to the patient's doctor or nursing home. Keep in mind that in an emergency, health-care providers do not need consent to treat patients, but must follow any known wishes of the patient with respect to treatment.

Each province handles this issue differently, and the hierarchy list for stand-in substitute decision-makers may not exist in every province and where it does exist, the list and rankings may not be the same across the country.

Communicate Care Directives

The second component of an advance care directive is communicating our care wishes, and expressing our values and beliefs to our appointed substitute decision-maker, other family members, and our family doctor.

Family conflicts may arise and create long-lasting tensions when a loved one's wishes are unknown. As well, tremendous anguish may result when family members are forced to make difficult medical treatment decisions for a parent or spouse who has not communicated his or her care directives.

Care instructions can be expressed orally, or can be in a written document. They can be part of the legal document that appoints our substitute decision-maker, or they can be in a separate document, called a Living Will or Health Care Directive. A Living Will is not a legal term in Ontario, but in some provinces there is a Health Care Directive that is a legal document.

Care directives that should be communicated to our substitute decision-maker are whether we want all medical heroics available to artificially keep us alive, if we are terminally ill, or to decline all artificial interventions, such as a feeding tube, a breathing ventilator, or resuscitation if our heart stops. Other topics that can be covered are organ donations when we die, blood transfusions, and specific treatments wanted or not wanted that are specific to our illnesses.

According to the Advocacy Centre for the Elderly in Toronto, "Our substitute decision-maker must follow our last known wishes when making decisions for us, when we are incapable, in accordance with the Health Care Consent Act. If they are not aware of any wishes applicable to the particular situation he or she must act in our best interests, and take into account our values and beliefs."[1]

While our substitute decision-maker must follow our expressed wishes, they have the tough job of interpreting them

---

[1] Advocacy Centre for the Elderly website, www.acelaw.ca, Advance Care Planning – Introduction.

and determining if they are applicable to the health-care decision that they are being asked to make. It is important to know that our care directives are only wishes, and cannot be used to provide instructions to our health-care providers, who must rely on our substitute decision-maker for direction based on our wishes, and for consent.

An aging adult should have a lawyer prepare the legal document to appoint a substitute decision-maker in the province where his or her care will be provided. Using a lawyer is also a good idea because they can provide legal advice specific to the individual's particular situation, and ensure that all the important directives have been included. Furthermore, they will be able to offer advice on the communication of care directives, and prepare Health Care Directive documents in the provinces where they are legal.

If hiring a lawyer is unaffordable, some provincial government websites have downloadable Power of Attorney kits that you can prepare yourself. Another option is to look for community legal clinics that provide free advice. Check under "legal aid" in the phone book. In Ontario, the Power of Attorney for Personal Care document must be prepared and signed by adults in front of two witnesses while they are mentally competent. They cannot be prepared and signed by family caregivers. There may be different witnessing requirements in other provinces.

MAKE FUNERAL ARRANGEMENTS

I raised the awkward topic of making advance funeral arrangements with my parents during a visit in the spring of 2001. Reluctantly, Mom decided to call a local funeral home to get a quote. My parents were uncomfortable saying the words *death, dying,* or *funeral,* so we jokingly started to substitute the word *MacCoubrey,* the name of the Cobourg funeral home they intended to use. I still remember my mother saying with a grin on her face, "I'm not ready for MacCoubrey yet," and my phone call to say, "I'm coming this weekend so we can discuss MacCoubrey." Finding lighter language made it easier for us to discuss their funeral arrangements.

I took Mom and Dad to visit cemeteries, and we openly discussed the options of a burial plot, or cremation with a niche in a columbarium. They chose cremation and a well-treed and well-kept cemetery, which was bordered on one side by a meandering brook and a golf course. My parents paid their chosen cemetery for a niche in a columbarium with an interment for both of them, which cost $1,600. At that time, they also decided on the lettering to appear on their niche.

Once those decisions were made, the three of us met with the funeral director to finalize their funeral arrangements. My parents decided that they would like a memorial service in the funeral home, and they designated their preferred charity, in lieu of flowers. They signed a service agreement with the funeral home for $4,600 per funeral. Then they purchased a group annuity for that amount, offered by a life insurance company. That gave them a guarantee that their financial obligations would be met, even if funeral prices increased by the time they died, if they moved and needed the services of a different funeral home, or if the funeral home went out of business.

In July 2001, my parents' funeral and burial arrangements were made and paid for. What started as an awkward conversation ended by taking a huge weight off their shoulders, and gave them a sense of peace. Dad died just 14 months later. My life would have been pure bedlam if we hadn't finished their funeral arrangements by then. Instead, the funeral director was just a phone call away, and he took care of everything, including my anxiety.

Some of the funeral arrangements that seniors and their family need to make include:

Cemetery

- which city or town
- which cemetery
- cremation or burial or some other option
- where in the cemetery

- wording on the tombstone or niche
- place ashes in a niche or scatter, and if the latter, where

Funeral

- which funeral home
- casket or urn
- choosing the pallbearers
- open or closed casket
- if open casket, in what clothes will the deceased be dressed
- visiting hours at funeral home
- newspaper notice
- type of service (memorial in church, funeral home, or other location)
- clergy or celebrant to officiate
- food for guests
- service at cemetery
- special requests for celebration of life

ESTABLISH THE FAMILY-CARE LEADERSHIP AND CAREGIVING TEAM IN WAITING

An advance care plan should be completed well before a parent or spouse needs care. The family member or members who have been appointed by parents or a spouse to be their Attorneys for Personal Care should become the family-care leaders. Their first decision should be to decide which of them would become the primary caregiver for a spouse, a surviving parent, or both parents if they need care at the same time. The primary caregiver usually is the person who lives closest to the elder or elders.

If family dynamics allow, the leaders should enlist other family members to form a caregiving team in waiting. This team should include the aging parents, other siblings, and their spouses and children. To solidify the family caregiving team, the care leaders and the aging parents should openly discuss the elements of the advance care plan, including appointments of Attorneys for Personal Care and end-of-life wishes, with all the caregiving team members.

It is important that the family caregiving team work as a cohesive unit, so they need to openly discuss, understand, and agree to their roles and responsibilities before they begin their care-team operations.

The 'family caregiving team in waiting' should then keep a watchful eye on their seniors, and be ready to start caregiving duties when they reach the supportive-living stage. At that juncture, the family-care leaders may be able to expand their team by adding close friends and neighbours who want to help. That would ensure the caregiving workload doesn't fall too heavily on the primary caregiver's shoulders for too long.

If an advance care plan is not undertaken and family members are unprepared for their responsibilities, they are likely to encounter a number of avoidable crises and hurdles during their caregiving journey. Accidents in the home, delays applying for a nursing-home placement, not knowing a loved one's end-of-life wishes, and having no funeral arrangements in place when they die are examples of crises and hurdles that may result in unnecessary stress, anguish, and workload for caregivers.

A lower standard of care and quality of life for an elder may be another one of the unfortunate consequences. If, however, parents miraculously die in their sleep, after a wonderfully healthy life, then the family caregiving team can put all their knowledge and planning skills to good use on their own end-of-life plans.

Once an advance care plan has been completed, family-care leaders should familiarize themselves with the living arrangement options and costs, so they can plan for the increasing financial demands of eldercare. This will help them ensure their loved ones obtain the best accommodations and care that they can afford.

TOP TIPS

Have Dialogue Early about Increasing Care Needs

- Discuss with seniors in their 70s, or earlier, their increasing care needs, and living arrangement options and preferences.
- Don't make promises you can't keep.

Encourage Early Preparations for End-of-Life

- Encourage seniors in their early 70s or sooner to:
  - legally appoint substitute decision-makers for personal care
  - communicate care directives to substitute decision-makers, other family members, and family doctor
  - express funeral arrangement wishes to family
  - make and pay for funeral and burial arrangements

Get a Head Start on Caregiving Responsibilities

- Become knowledgeable about the stages of elder decline and care needs at each stage.
- Establish 'family-care leadership and caregiving team in waiting.'

Keep a Watchful Eye

- Monitoring a senior's ability to perform the basic activities of daily life will help determine when a higher level of care is necessary.
- Look for warning signs of elder frailty that indicate when:
  - support needed to live independently in own home
  - unsafe to live alone
  - assistance needed with daily living

(5)

Financial Planning
for Senior Decline

My parents had very modest financial resources when they moved from Newfoundland to Ontario, where jobs were more plentiful in the 1940s. My father, a welder, found work in Toronto and was our family's sole breadwinner, and Mom stayed at home to raised David and me. My parents were very frugal, having been brought up in Newfoundland and having suffered through the hardship of the Great Depression. They were very resourceful at stretching Dad's hard-earned money, and despite their modest income, they saved for big purchases, a rainy day, and their retirement.

Once David and I got involved in handling our mother's financial affairs, we discovered that her annual accommodations and care costs surpassed her income. If we didn't manage her investments and expenses wisely, her money might run out if she lived ten more years.

To be successful, all businesses need to develop a good financial plan. The same is especially true for the business of eldercare because a senior's financial problems become a family's problems. A good financial plan will help ensure that family members understand the role they need to play in their loved one's financial security, a senior will receive the best quality of accommodations and care that they can afford, and costly mistakes will be avoided. The key components of a good financial plan include a money conversation with the family, estate planning, appointing of substitute decision-makers for property, succession planning, managing a senior's financial affairs, and forecasting how long a senior's money will last.

THE MONEY CONVERSATION WITH FAMILY

Families need to carefully plan for the time when a parent or spouse can no longer manage their own financial affairs, for the increasing financial demands of eldercare, and for the transfer of their capital assets and property when they die. Conversations about financial planning should happen when a senior is still healthy and able to discuss this issue objectively, ideally when they are in their 70s or earlier. To prevent family feuds, guilt, stress, or anxiety later on, all adult siblings and parents should be present for the money conversation.

Family members first need to make sure that aging loved ones have a will in place, so that the distribution of their capital assets and property will be carried out according to their wishes. It is important to know where the original signed will is kept. Each parent should by then also have legally appointed one or more substitute decision-makers to handle their financial affairs when they are unable to do so themselves.

Property insurance should also be discussed. Seniors will likely need to count on the equity in their home to help pay for their eldercare costs, so it will be reassuring to know that they have adequate insurance coverage. As with the will, it is important to know where these documents are kept.

Raise and resolve any family fears and concerns about whether or not parents have enough money to last until they die, and if they don't, whether adult children will pay for their parents' eldercare costs. If you have this candid conversation early, you can plan ahead. A very important question to address with all siblings and parents present is whether a son or daughter should consider giving up their job to care for a parent. If so, he or she needs to plan for their own financial security and whether other siblings are willing and able to help compensate for the financial loss.

As well, they need to know whether their parent, when they are of sound mind, would expect them to put their own retirement savings at risk. If they don't, this could save tremendous guilt later on when other care alternatives are being considered.

ESTATE PLANNING

Most people have an estate that includes capital assets, such as cash and investment securities; property, such as a house, a cottage, or a business; and possessions, such as a car, furniture, jewellery, and china. An estate includes both our assets and our liabilities, or debts, if we have any.

We all need to do estate planning to arrange for the transfer of everything that we own or have an interest in when we die to beneficiaries, such as a spouse, children, other relatives, business partners, charities, and other non-profit organizations. Determine what will be distributed as gifts during your life, and what will be distributed after your death. If an estate involves significant assets or complex issues, an estate-planning professional at a trust company or a lawyer can help prepare an estate plan.

I remember Mom's first forays into estate planning when she was in her 70s. She identified whom she wanted to give her cherished china and silverware keepsakes to by sticking their names on the bottom of each piece. If she had a lot of personal property to give away to many different people, it would have been better for her to attach a separate handwritten memorandum to her will. Unfortunately, in the stress and turmoil of clearing out my mother's house before she moved to a retirement residence, I lost sight of which of her prized possessions she wanted me to have. It wasn't until I read her will years later that I realized the significance of a Dutch windmill china figurine that had been in her family for generations. This was the only possession mentioned in her will and she named me as the beneficiary. Fortunately, she had given the precious ornament to my cousin Grace who graciously gave it to me.

The core element of any estate plan is the will, in which we appoint an estate trustee, also called an executor, a personal representative or a liquidator, who is responsible for carrying out the instructions in the will. He or she distributes the property to the beneficiaries, pays all of the deceased's debts and taxes, and completes the forms required by federal and provincial governments after our death.

Ideally, the estate trustee should be organized, impartial, reliable, and have some business experience. Once you've decided on someone, get their verbal agreement to take on this role before appointing them in your will, because it can be a time-consuming and sometimes complicated job. Also name a backup estate trustee in the will in case the person appointed is unable or unwilling to act on your behalf.

If you have no one willing or able to take this responsibility, you can appoint a trust company, an accountant, or a lawyer whose expertise and fees are acceptable. There is also an alternative: a provincial or territorial public trustee can be appointed as a last resort if a professional is unaffordable. If we die without a will, it is called dying *intestate*. Under the Succession Law Reform Act of all provinces and territories, the estate would be divided among our nearest relatives, using a formula that may differ somewhat by province.

We do not need to get legal advice to prepare a will, but it is prudent to do so since it is a legal document. Will kits and guides can help us get organized, but a lawyer experienced in estates can ensure that the document is prepared and witnessed correctly. In Quebec and B.C., a notary public can also prepare wills. It is a good idea to have your lawyer keep the original will and to keep a photocopy at home.

Keep your will up-to-date. If someone named in your will dies or there has been a divorce, remarriage, or birth in the family, you may need to make changes to reflect your current wishes.

APPOINTING SUBSTITUTE DECISION-MAKERS FOR PROPERTY

Any of us can find ourselves in a situation where we are temporarily or permanently too physically or mentally ill to handle our financial affairs. This can happen because of a stroke, cancer, dementia, an accident, or some other reason. Even if frail and ailing seniors are still mentally competent, they may have difficulty paying their bills, gathering receipts for their income tax return, managing their investments, and making decisions about their property. People with dementia are especially vulnerable.

An Enduring Power of Attorney, also called a Continuing Power of Attorney, is a legal document that gives us the ability to appoint one or more people as our attorney to manage our financial affairs. *Attorney*, in this instance, does not mean *lawyer*, but a substitute decision-maker. We should ask our prospective attorneys ahead of time, and they must accept the responsibility before they can be named. According to the Advocacy Centre for the Elderly (ACE) in Toronto, "depending on how the Power of Attorney is written, our attorney may have authority to: 1) act for us both when we are capable and when we are mentally incapable, or (2) act only when we have been found mentally incapable of managing our property and finances."[1]

If we choose the first option, our lawyer can retain the original document or we can keep it in a safety deposit box, until we decide we want our substitute decision-maker to take over our financial affairs. In 2000, Mom and Dad appointed David and me their attorneys while they were both mentally competent, but it was not until Dad died two years later that Mom asked us to manage her financial affairs.

If we don't have an Enduring or Continuing Power of Attorney in place and become mentally incapable of making decisions for ourselves, there are laws in every province and territory that allow the court to appoint a substitute decision-maker for us. This can, however, be a time-consuming and costly process for a family member or friend who is willing to take on the attorney role. As with a will, a lawyer should prepare the Enduring Power of Attorney to ensure we understand the risks and benefits of what we are signing. He or she will also make

---

[1] Advocacy Centre for the Elderly website, www.acelaw.ca, Powers of Attorney—Introduction.

certain that we meet the legal requirement of mental competency before preparing the document, and have two witnesses present for the signing.

Choose someone to be your substitute decision-maker who you have had a long-standing relationship with, who knows your wishes, and who you trust completely. The person should have high moral standards, and be good at handling money and making decisions. The only legal requirement is that they be 18 years of age or older.

If your financial affairs were fairly simple, a spouse, son, daughter, relative, or a good friend would be an appropriate person to ask; however, if your financial affairs are complicated, significant in value, or your spouse or children are uncomfortable taking over the reins, appoint a trust company to fill the substitute decision-maker role. Trust companies can pay bills and manage investments. Of course, they charge fees for these services. If this is unaffordable, as with a will, the public trustee, sometimes called the public guardian, can be appointed as a last resort.

It is a good idea to appoint two attorneys in the event that one named becomes incapable of acting, through death or incapacity, or is unavailable or unwilling to act when needed. Stipulate whether they must make decisions together or can act on their own, and include instructions for conflict resolution, such as one attorney's decisions always override the other, or a lawyer must resolve disputes.

David and I took our substitute decision-maker responsibility very seriously. We realized that it was not our money, but our parents' money that should be managed, and spent wisely on our mother. Dad would have expected no less from us. Only after our mother's needs had all been met and she had ascended into heaven, did we consider any residue money our inheritance.

Although attorneys are responsible for managing the incapacitated person's financial assets, they do not assume ownership of the property, income, or capital assets; that remains in the name of the senior. Similarly, attorneys are not personally liable for the senior's debts or other financial obligations. Attorneys for property are allowed to handle anything that the senior could handle, except to make or change their will. This includes opening and closing bank accounts; redirecting pensions and other income; applying for benefits or supplementary income to which the senior is entitled; choosing pension options; dealing with investments and income taxes; collecting and paying debts; paying bills; buying goods and services; selling, storing, and disposing of personal belongings; and maintaining or selling property.

The incapacitated person's financial accounts and transactions should be kept completely separate from the attorney's, who should never borrow or use the senior's money for themself. According to Ontario's Substitute Decisions Act, substitute decision-makers are legally obliged to keep complete and documented records of all their transactions, whether they involve the sale of the family house or paying a telephone bill. Other provinces likely have similar regulations. If attorneys don't keep good records, other family members may question how a loved one's money was spent. A lack of trust or confidence could lead to litigation or lifelong family feuds.

Once the senior dies, the Enduring Power of Attorney is null and void. According to the instructions in the will, authority to deal with the financial assets transfers immediately to the estate trustee.

SUCCESSION PLANNING

For many years my mother filed the family income tax return, but by her 70s she let David handle the job, and in her early 80s, she became so stressed out by her search for income tax receipts, she enlisted my help to sort out the mess and send David whatever he needed. We got the job done, but I'll never forget how upset Mom was. The following table lists warning signs of when a senior is having difficulty handling their financial affairs, and should start passing their financial baton to their substitute decision-makers for property.

Warning Signs that a Senior is Having Difficulty Handling Their Financial Affairs

Type of Difficulty	Warning Signs
Cognitive Problems	• Unopened and/or unpaid bills piling up • Confused about money matters
Stressed Out	• Upset by income tax returns
Eyesight & Hearing Problems	• Finding it hard to read bills • Having trouble hearing people
Lack of Initiative	• Lack of initiative in handling financial affairs
Disorganized	• No longer keeping good records and files
Physically Ill	• In hospital or care facility and too ill to handle finances
Can't Drive or Walk	• Can't get to the bank, grocery store, or mall

Once a senior has asked for help handling their financial affairs, learn their filing system and get as much information as soon as possible, before they possibly become incapacitated. This includes information about accounts with financial institutions, sources of income, health benefits, income tax returns, and insurance policies as well as contact information for any financial advisors. See the following table for a detailed list.

Financial Information Needed to Manage a Senior's Financial Affairs

Type of Information	Information Needed
Banking	• Bank accounts and credit cards, who has signing authority • Safety deposit box, location, box number, and key • Loans and mortgages, where held, account numbers
Investments	• Brokerage accounts, including RRSPs, RRIFs, and any annuities, which financial institutions, copy of statements, who has signing authority

Pensions & Other Sources of Income	• Old Age Security (OAS) Pension, and Canada Pension Plan (CPP) or Quebec Pension Plan (QPP) • Contacts and documents for employee, union, or veterans' pension • Rental and any other income
Health Benefits	• Employer, union, or veterans' benefits packages
Income Tax Returns	• Income tax returns for prior two years • File of current year receipts
Insurance	• House and automobile insurance policies • Health-care and long-term care insurance policies
Financial Advisors	• Contact information for investment advisor, financial planner, accountant, estate or trust company professional

The estate trustee of the will and the attorneys for personal care and property will need to know where to find information and legal documents relating to our will, funeral arrangements, property, life insurance, and other personal documents, such as marriage certificate and social insurance number. Contact information for our legal advisors will also be needed. See the following table for a detailed list of the estate information needed to administer a will. Most banks will provide their customers with an estate information organizer to list pertinent information and its location.

Estate Information Needed to Administer a Will

Type of Information	Information Needed
Funeral Arrangements	• Contract with funeral home for pre-arranged funeral • Funeral prepayment annuity document • Cemetery arrangement contract • Organ donation instructions *(Continued)*

Type of Information	Information Needed
Estate Plan	• Copy of will and location of original • List of personal possessions to be distributed • Estate trustee contact information • Copies of Power of Attorney documents for Personal Care and Property, and attorneys' contact information
Important Personal Documents	• Social insurance number • Birth and marriage certificates, marriage contract, any prenuptial agreements • Separation agreement or divorce decree • Health-insurance number and copy of card • Military service record and Veterans Affairs card
Property and Other Assets	• House and cottage deed and survey • Automobile ownership and registration • List of jewellery, stamp or coin collections, and other valuables
Life Insurance	• Insurance company name, policy number, beneficiary • Agent contact information
Legal Advisors	• Lawyer contact information for house ownership, will, and Power of Attorney documents

MANAGING A SENIOR'S FINANCIAL AFFAIRS

It may seem daunting at first to think of taking over your parents' or spouse's financial affairs, especially if you dislike handling your own finances. To help you get started, I have some tips I learned from running Doris Inc., which cover the following areas: taking over the management, record keeping and paying bills, investing, and completing income tax returns.

Taking Over Management

There are two ways that seniors can hand over the management of their financial affairs to someone else while they are still mentally capable. The first is to give their appointed substitute decision-makers for property a copy of their signed Enduring Power of Attorney. All financial institutions recognize the signing authority granted by this legal document, and they will keep a copy of it in their client's files. As described on page 82, ownership of bank and investment accounts remains in the senior's name, but substitute decision-makers have access and authority to use the accounts.

Seniors also have the option of changing their bank and investment accounts from single ownership (in their name only) to joint ownership with their attorney(s), or other person(s). If they have made that decision, they should indicate in the joint account agreement at the bank whether they grant their joint account owner(s) the *right of survivorship* or *no right of survivorship*. There is, however, no legal right of survivorship status available to joint account owners in Quebec, so citizens in that province must indicate no right of survivorship.

When a senior dies, joint account owner(s) who were granted right of survivorship are legally entitled to any funds in the financial institution accounts. These funds would essentially be removed from the senior's estate, and therefore not be subject to court probate process and fees. Probate provides legal validation that a will is not being contested, there is no other will in existence, and the estate trustees are the authorized executors of the will.

If a senior had chosen the joint ownership option with no right of survivorship, their accounts remain with their estate when they die. In that case, most financial institutions would not release funds to the joint account owner(s) or beneficiaries named in the will of the deceased without court probate verification.

While granting joint account owners the right of survivorship avoids probate court and fees, there is a significant downside to this option that may put the senior's estate at greater risk of financial abuse. If a joint account owner with right of survivorship status is unscrupulous, he or she could transfer all the assets to their own personal accounts, robbing other siblings and grandchildren, if there are any, of their rightful inheritance.

According to Doug Walker, a lawyer in Peterborough, Ontario, "this is such a common occurrence that the courts have taken a hard-line position. Without a joint account owner producing written proof from the deceased that he or she intended the financial assets to go to them, the court's assumption is that the assets belong to the estate, to be divided in accordance with the terms of the will."

Operating joint accounts with or without the right of survivorship can have a number of other unintended consequences, according to Alan Riccardi, manager, Estate & Trust Administration, at MD Private Trust Company. Joint account owners can:

- withdraw the senior's financial assets for their own use;
- expose the assets to their creditors or estranged spouse;
- create tax-reporting issues for the joint-account owners; and
- cause a lack of spending control because joint-account owners are not legally obliged to keep detailed records.

It would be wise for a senior to seek legal counsel before deciding how he or she will hand over the management of his or her financial affairs, because every family and financial situation is different. A lawyer can explain the unintentional consequences of each option, and draw up documents to clarify their intentions, which can be attached to their will. This should mitigate any future misunderstandings between the beneficiaries of the estate and the Canada Revenue Agency (CRA).

Record Keeping and Paying Bills

Keeping well-documented records of financial transactions needn't be difficult. First, use a banking record journal that you can buy at an office supply store to keep track of bill payments, automatic and cash withdrawals, and deposits. This information can also be kept on an Excel spreadsheet or some other financial-management software. It is important to record every cheque that you write and the reason for it. Also itemize any cash withdrawals you made, for example, to buy clothes and personal-care products, and keep the sales receipts in a separate file. The following table shows several examples of journal entries.

Example of Banking Record Journal Entries

Date	Cheque Made To	Cheque Number	Cheque Amount	✓	Deposit Amount	✓	Balance
June 1, 2011	Jenny Smith, caregiver-companion, 30 hours, May	20	$420.00	✓			$5,250.50
June 15	Bell Canada	21	45.25	✓			5,205.25
June 16	Cash withdrawal for personal-care products	cash	20.00				5,185.25
June 17	Canada Revenue Agency refund on income taxes				550.63	✓	5,735.88

To reduce the number of cheques that you have to write, set up automatic withdrawals for recurring monthly expenses, such as retirement residence fees, and telephone and television cable services. It is also a good idea to arrange for bills to be sent to your home address once your loved one is no longer living in their own home.

David and I kept a tight rein on expenses to ensure that Mom's money wasn't wasted, and agreed to discuss any expense over $150. If we didn't agree, we found some other solution to meet Mom's needs. This arrangement works well if there is more than one substitute decision-maker handling a senior's financial affairs. Using on-line banking to keep an eye on the bank balance also makes sense, so that you won't be overdrawn.

Investing a Senior's Money

When my mother moved into a retirement residence, David invested the proceeds from the sale of her house. He also switched her invested capital assets from low-interest-bearing bonds and guaranteed investment certificates (GICs) to higher-income-generating investments to help pay for her expenses. Mom was glad to have him managing her investments because he is a Chartered Accountant and investment advisor with a major Canadian investment firm.

My brother's investment objectives were to diversify her capital assets, and choose slightly higher yielding yet still fairly secure securities that would improve income. He was well aware that seniors have a greater need for income and a lower tolerance for risk than younger people. He monitored her investments often and was able to generate, on average, a 5 per cent return each year.

Managing a senior's investments can be more difficult than for a younger investor, because the value of investments can rise or fall dramatically in a short period of time. If $100,000 in capital assets are lost in the early stage of a senior's decline, they may not recover the funds in time to pay for all of their eldercare expenses. Their money must, therefore, be conservatively invested. A 4 to 6 per cent return range is a high enough goal to set, because securities that promise a higher return usually come with a higher risk.

If you do not have the financial expertise or the time to manage your loved one's capital assets, then seeking professional help makes sense, but it can also be confusing as there are many different types: investment advisors, financial advisors, financial planners, investment specialists, financial consultants, and life insurance underwriters. They don't all offer the same range of services, and they are not all licensed to sell the same types of financial products. Families need to ensure they are comfortable with the products an advisor is selling, and the associated risk, before they put them on their short list of potential candidates.

There are three investment advisor designations to look for that will help in the selection process: a certified senior advisor (CSA) who has been trained in how to invest for the 55-plus age group, certified financial planner (CFP), and chartered accountant (CA), as well as a business degree, are all good indications that an investment advisor has strong financial expertise.

It is a good idea to find an older and experienced advisor who will likely relate well and have more empathy for a senior's situation. It also makes sense to specify in writing that your investment goal is to generate income to pay for eldercare costs and to keep risk low.

My brother recommends interviewing three financial advisors, asking for two references from each, and then assessing the qualifications, experience, and performance record of each. Visit the Investment Industry Regulatory Organization of Canada (www.iiroc.ca) and the Ontario Securities Commission (www. getsmarteraboutmoney.ca) websites for advice and questions to ask when choosing an investment advisor.

Completing Income Tax Returns

Filing income tax returns can be complicated, so consider hiring an accountant or service to complete this task. Depending on the complexity, accountants usually charge $100 to $300 to complete and file a return electronically to the Canada Revenue Agency (CRA).

For many seniors, it won't be expensive. This option will save you time, he or she will usually answer all kinds of tax-related questions, and keep an ongoing file for you. There are a number of exemptions, deductions, and tax credits that can lower a senior's tax burden. For more information, visit the CRA website (www.cra.gc.ca) or call 1-800-959-8281.

Regardless of who does the tax return, it is important for you to keep good records of your loved one's tax-deductible expenses, including receipts for medical expenses, hearing-aid insurance, charitable donations, as well as statements of annual income from financial institutions and pension companies, such as T3s, T4s, T5s, etc. I kept a file of all these receipts and at the end of March each year I sent copies to my brother, along with a copy of the banking record journal for the prior year, so he had the information he needed to complete our mother's tax return.

FORECASTING HOW LONG A SENIOR'S MONEY WILL LAST

The biggest question David and I faced when we started to manage our mother's financial affairs was whether she would likely run out of money before she died. We specifically needed to know how long her income and capital assets would cover the cost of her accommodations, and the level of care that we wanted for her.

Accountants use a financial planning tool called a *capital depletion forecast* to answer this question. Capital is the money and property owned by a senior that can be used to earn income and pay for their eldercare expenses. The forecast keeps track of the estimated inflows and outflows of money and the cash available to pay bills each year. Whenever spending exceeds income for a year, the capital will be reduced. Ultimately, this planning tool estimates when a senior's money is likely to run out.

With a good sense of available financial resources, families can develop an affordable care plan that will meet the needs of their loved one, by adopting one of the following three care strategies:

Significant Financial Resources

• Confidently spend to provide the best care possible because money is unlikely to run out.

Moderate Financial Resources

• Spend cautiously, attempt to improve the income on investments, and take advantage of any available tax deductions and credits, so that a senior can have a good level of care that lasts as long as they are likely to live.

Very Limited Financial Resources

• Seek government-subsidized accommodations and care, as well as community-based low-cost and volunteer support if a senior is likely to run out of money very soon. Provide more family care and plan for how any shortfall will be covered.

Capital assets, income, income taxes, spending, and the forecast period are the five inputs needed to create a capital depletion forecast. The following is a simplified numeric example of the capital depletion calculations that are needed for every year of the forecast period:

Simplified Capital Depletion Forecast for Year 1

Annual Income	$22,000		
Less Income Taxes	2,000		
Disposable Income	20,000		
Less Annual Spending	−40,000	**Beginning Capital Assets**	**$100,000**
Capital Depletion	**$20,000** ➜	**Less Capital Depletion**	**−20,000**
		Capital Assets End of Year	**$ 80,000**

Annual income and spending are the most important inputs in a capital depletion forecast because they determine whether a senior's capital assets will grow or decline each year. They also determine how long the capital assets will last. If a senior is fortunate to have higher income than spending, their capital will grow, so they will not run out of money before they die.

In the more common scenario, a senior will have higher accommodations and care costs, living expenses, and discretionary spending than income, so the amount of capital will decline each year. One of the consequences of declining capital is shrinking investment income, because he or she will have less money to invest in each subsequent year. As time goes on, this will widen the gap between expenses and income, and accelerate the rate of capital depletion. It is therefore important to keep track of how fast your loved one's money is being depleted.

Here is a step-by-step guide to completing a capital depletion forecast that explains what should be included in capital assets, annual income, annual spending, and the forecast period.

Step 1: Determine Capital Assets

Capital assets are investments, such as stocks, bonds, debentures, GICs, income trusts, mutual funds, and cash in the bank. Include the equity in the home and any other property, such as a cottage, that could be sold and the net proceeds invested to earn income to pay for eldercare costs. Subtract loans or mortgages on property from the total capital.

When we took over managing Mom's money she had a total of $400,000 in capital assets, $250,000 in fixed-income securities (mostly government bonds and GICs), and $150,000 in cash from the sale of our parent's small brick bungalow. This was our starting point for planning purposes.

Step 2: Identify Sources of Annual Income

Income typically comes from pension sources, such as the Old Age Security (OAS) program and the Canada Pension Plan (CPP) or Quebec Pension Plan (QPP). Seniors with low income may also qualify for a Guaranteed Income Supplement (GIS). Employer, union, or veterans' pensions are other sources of income.

There may also be investment income that can include interest, dividends, and distributions earned on cash in bank accounts, and stocks, bonds, debentures, income trusts, mutual funds, annuities, and GICs. Most often, these investments are held in a Registered Retirement Savings Plan (RRSP), which is usually converted to a Registered Retirement Income Fund (RRIF) once a senior reaches the age of 71. A percentage of the capital in a RRIF is paid out each year.

Mom's annual income was $39,500, half from pensions and annuities and half from investments. She received $19,500 per year, or $1,625 a month, from pensions and two annuities: $148 from Dad's union pension trust fund, $473 from OAS, $474 from Dad's CPP, and $530 from two annuities. In the first year he managed her money, David earned $20,000 in investment income on Mom's $400,000 in capital assets, which included the proceeds from the sale of her house.

Step 3: Forecast Annual Spending as Health Declines

Accommodations and care are the biggest expenses, and are available at "economy-," "business-," and "first-class" prices, in the same way that you can buy airline tickets for different seats with correspondingly different prices. Chart #1 below shows two scenarios with estimates of typical eldercare spending. Scenario A includes a lower level of spending for a senior with lower-middle-class means. Scenario B has medium-level spending for a senior with middle-class resources. I did not include a high spending level because there would be only a small percentage of wealthy seniors who could afford a first-class level of spending.

The spending forecasts cover accommodations and care estimates for commonly used living arrangements, moving from a retirement residence, into an assisted-living residence, and then into a nursing home as a senior's health declines. A broader range of accommodations and care alternatives, cost ranges, and cost comparisons, including the option of providing care at home, are covered in chapter 8.

The spending forecasts also include lower and medium estimates for other living expenses that elders will typically incur, such as utilities, assistive devices, clothes and footwear, personal-care products and services, medical expenses, transportation, spending money, and a contingency fund for unexpected expenses.

Annual Eldercare Spending Estimates: Chart #1

Spending Category	Description of Spending	Scenario A	Scenario B
A. Accommodations & Care	• Retirement residence	$30,000	$48,000
	• Assisted-living residence	$42,000	$60,000
	• Nursing home (Ontario fees included)	$19,500	$26,000
B. Other Living Expenses Utilities	• Telephone and cable TV. Expenses may or may not be included in seniors' residence fees	$800	$1,200
Assistive Devices	• Hearing aids, mobility aids, wheelchair, walker, oxygen, prostheses, etc., whatever portion isn't paid by provincial government • Insurance, batteries and repairs on hearing aids	$700	$1,200
Clothes & Footwear	• Regular and specialty clothing	$800	$1,500
Personal-Care Products & Services	• Toiletries, haircuts, manicures	$400	$600
Medical Expenses	• Dental and eye care, eyeglasses, foot care • Medications and physiotherapy not covered by provincial government	$600	$1,300

Transportation	• Taxis to medical appointments • Special buses that provide wheelchair access • Emergency and non-emergency ambulances	$200	$600
Spending Money	• Gifts, donations, personal spending	$200	$1,000
Contingency Fund	• Reserve for unexpected expenses	$300	$600
Total Other Living Expenses		$4,000	$8,000
C. Caregiver-Companions	• Retirement residence	$0	$0
	• Assisted living: Scenario B 2 hrs/day	$0	$13,000
	• Nursing home: Scenario A 2 hrs/day Scenario B 4 hrs/day	$13,000	$26,000
Total Annual	**Retirement residence**	**$34,000**	**$56,000**
Spending Estimate	**Assisted-living residence**	**$46,000**	**$81,000**
(Total A+B+C Above)	**Nursing home**	**$36,500**	**$60,000**

In the assisted-living residence estimate, I built in two hours a day of caregiver-companion support in the medium-spending scenario. This would be quite helpful because by then many seniors have only a limited ability to socialize. In the nursing home estimate, I built in four hours a day of caregiver-companion support in the medium-spending scenario, and two hours a day in the lower-spending scenario. Once seniors reach the dependent-living stage in a nursing home, they can all benefit greatly from caregiver-companion attention and care. Your capital depletion schedule will determine if this discretionary expense is affordable.

If hiring privately, families should budget for caregiver-companions at $18 an hour as I did in Chart #1, although they may be able to obtain help at a lower hourly rate. If hiring through an agency, families should plan to pay at least $22 an hour for companions, and $28 an hour for personal support workers when more care than companionship is required. These rates will vary by province, and by urban versus rural areas.

Chart #3 on page 106 provides a 10-year forecast based on annual eldercare spending estimates from Chart #1, for Scenarios A and B. The projections are available by retirement residences, assisted-living residences, and nursing homes, and include accommodations and care costs, other living expenses, and caregiver-companion support. A 2 per cent inflation factor has been added in years 2 to 10 so spending forecasts will cover any cost-of-living increases, which is realistic in today's economic environment.

These spending forecasts will help you develop a plan for your loved one's situation. These projections assume seniors are likely to need to move to a residence with care support of some kind as their health declines, and some will need all three types of facilities. If he or she is already living in an assisted-living facility, your forecast should begin with the assisted-living spending estimate in year 1, and then later switch to the nursing-home spending estimates, for example, starting in year 4.

Step 4: Predict Forecast Period

The capital depletion forecast period will depend on the senior's age and health; whether they have reached the supportive-, assisted-, or dependent-living stage of decline; and the severity, complexity, and predictability of their illnesses. When we took over managing Mom's finances, she exhibited early signs of Alzheimer's disease, which on average lasts for 8 to 12 years. She was already 84, so we felt that planning for 10 years of eldercare expenses would be plenty.

Step 5: Complete Capital Depletion Forecast

To complete a capital depletion forecast, look at the Doris Inc. Capital Depletion Forecasts for Scenarios A and B on pages 107–110, in Charts #4 and #5, and then follow the instructions below.

Forecast Period

Choose the forecast period, such as 5, 10, or 15 years, that best reflects how long you think your loved one will likely live. This will determine how long to run your capital depletion forecast.

Capital Depletion Forecast

Copy the spreadsheet format of the Doris Inc. Capital Depletion Forecast into Microsoft Excel or another financial-management computer software, or download Chart #4 or #5 from John Wiley & Sons Canada's website (http://ca.wiley.com/WileyCDA search for Doris Inc.). Then enter the following data, using Chart #2 on pages 100–101 as a guide.

① Senior's beginning capital assets in year 1.

② Estimated rate of return on investments, such as 4, 5, or 6 per cent.

③ Pensions and other income for year 1. Add a cost-of-living factor such as 2 per cent in year 2 and onward, if appropriate.

④ Current-year federal and provincial income tax rates, obtained from the Canada Revenue Agency's website, www.cra.gc.ca.

⑤ Tax credits, exemptions, and deductions.

⑥ Spending forecast for year 1 to end of forecast period, adjusted by cost-of-living factor for year 2 and onward. Use Chart #3, entitled "10-Year Eldercare Spending Forecast for Scenarios A and B," on page 106 as a guide.

Plug in adding, subtracting, and multiplying formulas into the spreadsheet software, using Chart #2 as a guide. If you download a Doris Inc. Capital Depletion Forecast for Scenario A or B, Chart #4 or #5, from the John Wiley & Sons Canada's website, then the mathematical formulae will already be imbedded in your spreadsheets.

Capital Depletion Forecast Methodology Explained
(Calculations by Line for Scenario B)

Chart #2

Line Item	Explanation	Year 1	Year 2
① **Capital Assets Beginning of Year**	• Investments, cash in bank accounts and equity in a home that can be sold and invested to pay eldercare costs • Subtract any debts from total capital assets	$400,000	$376,184
② Income % Return on Investment Income	• Estimated rate of income on invested money (i.e., bonds, stocks, debentures, income trusts, GICs, mutual funds)	4%	4%
② Income Investment Income on Capital Assets	• Estimated 4% rate of return multiplied by beginning of year capital	16,000	15,047
③ Federal Government Pension Income	• OAS and CPP, including a 2% cost-of-living factor, in years 2 to 10	12,300	12,546
③ Other Pensions & Income	• Company pensions, annuities, and income from other sources: a cost-of-living factor may or may not apply	8,000	8,000
Total Income before Taxes	• Sum of investment income, government and other pensions, and other income sources	36,300	35,593
④ Federal & Provincial Taxes	• Multiply income before taxes by federal plus provincial tax rates (20% in Ontario for 2011) • Tax rates will depend on senior's income bracket and will likely change each year	7,260	7,119

(Continued)

Capital Depletion Forecast Methodology Explained (Calculations by Line for Scenario B)   Chart #2

Line Item	Explanation	Year 1	Year 2
⑤ Tax Credits, Exemptions, and Deductions	• Federal basic personal ($10,527) and age tax credits ($6,036) for person over 65 with an income of $36,300 in 2011 were $16,563, multiplied by federal tax rate of 15% = $2,484; plus, Ontario basic personal ($9,104) and age tax credits $3,944 were $13,048, multiplied by Ontario tax rate of 5.05% = $660	3,144	3,144
	Note: If net income exceeds a threshold amount the age tax credit is reduced or even eliminated.		
	• Other deductions and tax credits may reduce taxes further		
Taxes Payable	• Federal and provincial taxes less tax credits, exemptions, and deductions	4,116	$3,974
Disposable Income after Taxes	• Total income before taxes minus taxes payable	32,184	31,619
⑥ Spending Adjusted for Cost of Living	• Eldercare spending forecast, using Chart #3 as a guide	56,000	57,120
Capital Depletion	• Annual spending minus disposable income after taxes that yields a negative balance	−23,816	−25,501
	• If disposable income after taxes is greater than expenses, then capital appreciation rather than depreciation occurs		
Capital Assets End of Year	• Capital assets at beginning of year *less* capital depletion, or *plus* capital appreciation	**$376,184**	**$350,683**

The beauty of using Excel or another financial-management software is that families will be able to insert various spending alternatives, and then see what impact they have on how long their loved one's money will last. As well, if a senior's circumstances and costs change, families will be able to input new numbers and the mathematical formulas will automatically recalculate their totals, and revise their forecast.

Families may feel more comfortable having an accountant or investment advisor complete their capital depletion forecast; however, the starting capital assets, annual income, spending forecast and forecast period will need to be provided to an accountant or financial advisor, in order for them to complete their capital depletion forecast.

Capital Depletion Forecasts for Scenarios A and B

Capital depletion forecasts for Scenarios A and B are on page 107–110 in Charts #4 and #5. They compare how long a senior's money would last with lower and medium levels of capital assets, income and eldercare spending. In Scenario A, the senior has starting capital assets of $200,000, and in Scenario B $400,000. In both cases, the forecasts run for ten years and assume the seniors live for three years in a retirement residence, two years in an assisted-living facility, and then five years in a nursing home.

Scenario A: Senior with $200,000 in Capital Assets, Plus Lower Income and Spending

The senior in Scenario A can afford to move into a small but private apartment in a retirement residence for three years, a small but private assisted-living apartment for two years and then into a shared room in a nursing home for three years, before they would likely run out of money in year nine. They could afford to pay for two hours a day of caregiver-companion support for their first three years in a nursing home. After that, their family and volunteers would need to provide the extra care and companionship.

In order for the money to last eight years, a 4 per cent investment return on capital assets would have to be achieved, and the senior would need to receive the average CPP and OAS benefit of $12,300 a year in 2011.

Scenario B: Senior with $400,000 in Capital Assets, Plus Medium Income and Spending

The senior with $400,000 in capital assets would receive good care for nine years with a medium income and spending level, before their money would likely run out in year 10. He or she could afford two hours a day of caregiver-companion support while in an assisted-living residence, and four hours a day for four years in a nursing home.

This scenario assumes the choice of a larger apartment in retirement and assisted-living residences and a private room in a nursing home, compared to the senior in Scenario A. It also assumes the senior would have additional income of $8,000 a year, beyond the $12,300 in government pensions.

Surprisingly, the senior in Scenario A with $200,000 in capital assets could afford to pay for a good level of care that would last for eight years, only one year less than the senior with $400,000 in capital assets. With the help of this financial-planning tool, family-care leaders can get the guidance they need to ensure their loved one receives the best accommodations and care that they can afford for as long as possible. In both scenarios, the capital depletion forecast provides enough advance warning to apply for a government subsidy of nursing-home costs for any additional years that the senior lived.

Doris Inc. had a good financial plan and David and I worked well as a team to invest and manage our mother's money, and to buy her whatever she needed. Our capital depletion forecast gave us the confidence to significantly increase our spending on her caregiver-companions as her health declined, because we knew she was unlikely to outlive her capital assets. The end result was good care for Mom, and we still had lives of our own.

TOP TIPS

Have a Family Conversation Early about Financial Matters

- Family members need to have a frank conversation with their aging loved ones, when they are in their 70s or sooner, to discuss how they will handle their increasing financial and care needs.

Ensure Seniors' Financial Ducks Are in a Row

- Encourage seniors when they are in their 70s or sooner to:
  - prepare a will;
  - appoint a substitute decision-maker to handle their financial affairs when they can no longer do so;
  - confirm they have adequate property insurance; and
  - prepare a financial and estate information organizer for whomever will manage their affairs.

A Good Financial Plan Creates Family Harmony

- Seniors' financial problems become family financial problems.
- A good financial plan helps to ensure that:
  - senior's financial wishes will be carried out;
  - family members understand the role they need to play in a seniors' financial security; and
  - seniors receive the best accommodations and care that they can afford.

Invest Senior's Money Conservatively

- Seniors have a greater need for income and a lower tolerance for risk than younger people.

Money is Your Friend

- Use a capital depletion forecast to obtain a good sense of a senior's available financial resources in future years. This financial tool will help families develop an afford-able care plan that will meet their loved one's needs for as long as they live.

10-Year Eldercare Spending Forecast for Scenarios A and B										Chart #3
Forecasts by Accommodations and Care Options (Canadian costs)										
	Year 1	Year 2	Year 3	Year 4	Year 5	Year 6	Year 7	Year 8	Year 9	Year 10
Retirement Residence										
Scenario A	34,000	34,680	35,374	36,081	36,803	37,539	38,290	39,055	39,836	40,633
Scenario B	56,000	57,120	58,262	59,428	60,616	61,829	63,065	64,326	65,613	66,925
Assisted-Living Residence										
Scenario A	46,000	46,920	47,858	48,816	49,792	50,788	51,803	52,840	53,896	54,974
Scenario B	81,000	82,620	84,272	85,958	87,677	89,431	91,219	93,044	94,904	96,802
Includes caregiver-companions for 2 hrs/day										
Nursing Home										
Scenario A	36,500	37,230	37,975	38,734	39,509	40,299	41,105	41,927	42,766	43,621
Includes caregiver-companions for 2 hrs/day										
Scenario B	60,000	61,200	62,424	63,672	64,946	66,245	67,570	68,921	70,300	71,706
Includes caregiver-companions for 4 hrs/day										

Notes:

Scenario A: lower spending estimate; Scenario B: medium spending estimate

Spending forecasts include: accommodations and care costs by type of seniors' residence; other living expenses and spending on caregiver-companions

Spending has been adjusted for a 2% cost-of-living factor in years 2–10.

Cost estimates in year 1 are based on available mid-2010 to mid-2011 data.

Doris Inc. Capital Depletion Forecast for Scenario A

Based on $200,000 in Capital Assets & Lower Income and Spending Level

(Canadian dollars, 2011 federal and Ontario tax structure)

Chart #4

| | Retirement Residence | | | Assisted-Living Residence | | Nursing Home | | | | |
	Year 1	Year 2	Year 3	Year 4	Year 5	Year 6	Year 7	Year 8	Year 9	Year 10
Capital Assets Beginning of Year	200,000	185,484	170,020	153,568	123,352	91,402	68,136	43,537	17,550	−10,103
Income										
% Return on Investment Income	4%	4%	4%	4%	4%	4%	4%	4%	4%	4%
Investment Income on Capital Assets	8,000	7,419	6,801	6,143	4,934	3,656	2,725	1,741	702	0
Government Pension Income Indexed for Inflation @ 2% starting in year 2*	12,300	12,546	12,797	13,053	13,314	13,580	13,852	14,129	14,411	14,700
Other Pensions & Income	0	0	0	0	0	0	0	0	0	0
Total Income Before Taxes	20,300	19,965	19,598	19,196	18,248	17,236	16,577	15,870	15,113	14,700

(Continued)

Taxes									
Federal & Provincial Taxes 20%**	4,060	3,993	3,920	3,839	3,650	3,447	3,315	3,174	3,023	2,940
Less Basic Personal & Age Tax Credits***	3,244	3,244	3,244	3,244	3,244	3,244	3,244	3,244	3,244	3,244
Fed. & Prov. Taxes Payable****	816	749	676	595	406	203	72	−70	0	0
Disposable Income after Taxes	19,484	19,216	18,922	18,600	17,842	17,033	16,506	15,940	15,113	14,700
Spending Adjusted for Cost of Living	34,000	34,680	35,374	48,816	49,792	40,299	41,105	41,927	42,766	43,621
Capital Depletion										
Disposable Income Spending Less	14,516	15,464	16,452	30,216	31,950	23,266	24,599	25,987	27,653	28,921
Capital Assets End of Year	185,484	170,020	153,568	123,352	91,402	68,136	43,537	17,550	−10,103	−39,024

Assumptions:

*Average Canada Pension Plan ($6,000), and maximum Old Age Security benefit ($6,300) paid in 2011 = $12,300.

**Tax rates used are the 2011 federal rate of 15% for income under $42,000, combined with 5.05% Ontario tax rate for income under $38,000.

***Federal basic personal ($10,527) & age tax credits ($6,537 for person over 65 with income under $32,961) were $17,064 multiplied by federal tax rate of 15% = $2,560, plus Ontario basic personal ($9,104) and age tax credits ($4,445) were $13,549 multiplied by the Ontario tax credit of 5.05% = $684. Other deductions & tax credits may reduce an elder's income further. Tax credits will vary by year and province.

****If taxes payable are a negative number, taxes payable are 0.

Doris Inc. Capital Depletion Forecast for Scenario B　　Chart #5

Based on $400,000 in Capital Assets & Medium Income and Spending Level

(Canadian dollars, 2011 federal and Ontario tax structure)

	Retirement Residence			Assisted-Living Residence		Nursing Home				
	Year 1	Year 2	Year 3	Year 4	Year 5	Year 6	Year 7	Year 8	Year 9	Year 10
Capital Assets Beginning of Year	400,000	376,184	350,683	323,435	267,814	208,902	169,751	128,239	84,269	37,739
Income										
% Return on Investment Income	4%	4%	4%	4%	4%	4%	4%	4%	4%	4%
Investment Income on Capital Assets	16,000	15,047	14,027	12,937	10,713	8,356	6,790	5,130	3,371	1,510
Government Pension Income Indexed for Inflation @ 2%*	12,300	12,546	12,797	13,053	13,314	13,580	13,852	14,129	14,411	14,700
Other Pensions & Income	8,000	8,000	8,000	8,000	8,000	8,000	8,000	8,000	8,000	8,000
Total Income Before Taxes	**36,300**	**35,593**	**34,824**	**33,990**	**32,026**	**29,936**	**28,642**	**27,258**	**25,782**	**24,209**

(Continued)

Taxes										
Federal & Provincial Taxes 20%**	7,260	7,119	6,965	6,798	6,405	5,987	5,728	5,452	5,156	4,842
Less Basic Personal & Age Tax Credits***	3,144	3,144	3,144	3,144	3,144	3,144	3,144	3,144	3,144	3,144
Fed. & Prov. Taxes Payable**	4,116	3,974	3,820	3,654	3,261	2,843	2,584	2,307	2,012	1,697
Disposable Income after Taxes	32,184	31,619	31,004	30,337	28,766	27,093	26,058	24,951	23,770	22,512
Spending Adjusted for Cost of Living	56,000	57,120	58,252	85,958	87,677	66,245	67,570	68,921	70,300	71,706
Capital Depletion										
Spending Less Disposable Income	23,816	25,501	27,248	55,621	58,911	39,152	41,512	43,970	46,530	49,194
Capital Assets End of Year	376,184	350,683	323,435	267,814	208,902	169,751	128,239	84,269	37,739	−11,455

Assumptions:

*Average Canada Pension Plan ($6,000), and maximum Old Age Security benefit ($6,300) paid in 2011 = $12,300.

**Tax rates used are the 2011 federal rate of 15% for income under $42,000, combined with 5.05% Ontario tax rate for income under $38,000.

***Federal basic personal ($10,527) & age tax credits ($6,036 for person over 65 with $36,300 in income) were $16,563 multiplied by federal tax rate of 15% = $2,484, plus. Ontario basic personal ($9,104) & age tax credits ($3,944) were $13,048 multiplied by the Ontario tax rate of 5.05% = $660. Other deductions & tax credits may reduce an elder's income further. Tax credits will vary by year and province.

****If taxes payable are a negative number, taxes payable are 0.

(6)

Elder Proofing to Reduce Preventable Crises

A fall is often a life-changing event for seniors, especially if it results in a hip, spine, or leg fracture, or a head injury. It can mean the end of independent living, a long rehabilitation, for some a sharp decline in mental capabilities, a move into a nursing home, or even death. A serious fall can also mean an early and abrupt start to caregiving duties, with an accelerated introduction to the myriad of health-care professionals and suppliers who specialize in eldercare.

As physical and sometimes mental capabilities erode with age, people are more vulnerable to accidents that can cause injury and a sudden decline in health. Seniors are slower to heal and have more mobility problems than younger people. They are also more likely to have an adverse complication from medications, surgeries, and medical devices. Fortunately, some of these common crises are predictable and preventable.

Elder proofing makes an environment safer for aging adults so they avoid unnecessary pain and suffering, and can live independently longer. Mom and Dad would have been horrified by the term *elder proofing*, but that was exactly what we started to do when they were in their late 70s and entering the supportive-living stage of decline.

Of course, my brother and I couldn't protect our parents from all accidents, but we worked with them to implement several initiatives that kept them safe for many years. Our elder-proofing initiatives fell into two categories: building a safety net so that they had ready access to help when needed, and reducing their risk of common preventable accidents that typically happen to older people.

BUILD A SAFETY NET

What would happen if your aging parent fell down a flight of stairs and was knocked unconscious, or had a stroke when they were alone in their house? How would your mother or father get emergency help? How would you feel if you couldn't reach your parent several times on a day when you expected them to be home? Where would you turn for help to determine if they were in danger?

Having a safety net in place for seniors before a life-threatening emergency occurs ensures that they have immediate access to medical attention, which can prevent catastrophes, such as a person not being found for days. A safety net reduces complications by getting them the help they need quickly, while at the same time providing peace of mind to all family members.

Seniors also need ready access to assistance when they have questions or concerns, or are unable to handle a problem on their own. Finding a neighbour to do odd jobs around the house, such as replacing a light bulb in a ceiling light fixture, can prevent a fall and injury, which is especially important when a senior lives alone.

For Christmas one year, I bought my parents a phone specially designed for declining vision and hearing abilities; it had big numbers, a memory of the most important phone numbers, a loud ringer, a volume amplifier that would make a caller's voice louder, and a light that would flash when the phone rang. I entered the phone numbers of key people who would be part of my parents' safety net into the phone memory including me, my brother, their neighbour across the street, and Mom's friend

Sue, who would come if either of them didn't feel well. My parents could then just press a button rather than dial a phone number to reach one of us. Mom and Dad also had a cordless phone that they could take outside while they were gardening so they wouldn't feel they had to run for the phone in the house for fear of missing an important call.

I also compiled a phone directory with large type on my computer that I printed and put in a bright green binder so my parents had easy access to all the important people and organizations in their lives, arranged under the following headings: emergencies, medical specialists, relatives, friends and neighbours, and businesses. David and I had a copy of the phone directory too, so we had access to neighbours whom we could call if we couldn't reach Mom and Dad.

My parents had already given David and me keys to their house many years earlier, but in their 70s they decided to give copies to a few trusted neighbours as well. That way, in an emergency a neighbour could easily get into the house.

A MedicAlert bracelet is another good safety-net initiative that can save lives, if a senior has allergies or a medical condition that puts them at risk in an emergency. For a small annual fee, people can wear a MedicAlert bracelet bearing an identification number that emergency medical personnel use when they call the organization's 24-hour emergency hotline, to find out the person's pre-existing medical problems.

After my father died, I encouraged my mother to let me install a 24-hour-a-day personal emergency-response system in her home. I searched "personal medical alert" on the Internet and found several well-established companies. Mom and I chose one that would install the equipment free of charge in the Cobourg area. The company charged a small monthly fee and the service could be cancelled at any time.

The medical alert system works this way: A help button is embedded in a waterproof bracelet, pendant, or belt clip that is worn by a person around their home at all times. If he or she needs medical assistance, they push the button and it connects wirelessly to a two-way voice communicator unit, which is installed beside a phone in a central location of the home. A medical alert signal is sent to the monitoring centre of the emergency response company. Using the two-way communicator, an operator immediately tries to speak to the person and ask him or her if they are all right. If the person needs medical assistance or if they can't speak, the operator dispatches an ambulance and notifies a designated neighbour, friend, or family member so they can open the door for the ambulance drivers.

One night, Mom unintentionally tested her new personal emergency-response system. She was sleeping very soundly, when suddenly she felt a hand gently nudging her shoulder. In total shock and disbelief, she saw her neighbour standing over her and two young ambulance drivers at the foot of her bed staring down at her. She had accidentally knocked the pendant off her night table, and when it hit the hardwood floor the help button was activated. She always removed her two hearing aids when she slept so she couldn't hear the operator's voice from the living room phone. If nothing else, we certainly found out just how valuable and reliable this type of service can be in a real emergency, and we had a few laughs when we recounted the story.

REDUCE COMMON PREVENTABLE ACCIDENTS

Falls, adverse drug reactions, and hospital-acquired infections are three of the most common accidents that happen to older people. Elder-proofing initiatives can reduce the risk of these mishaps by proactively eliminating the typical causes of each accident.

Reduce the Risk of a Fall and Injury

My parents' perceptual awareness started to decline when they were in their early 70s, as their vision and hearing abilities deteriorated with age. Their reflexes and balance weren't as good either. By then, their joints became stiffer, and they had lost a good deal of the muscle and bone mass that they had in their youth. These diminishing physical capabilities put my parents, and many other older adults, at an increased risk of a fall because they were less stable on their feet. Seniors are also at a higher risk of falling if they have had a fall before, have Parkinson's disease, osteoporosis, dementia, arthritis, multiple chronic illnesses, a vision impairment, have suffered a stroke, or are heavily medicated.

Sleeping pills can increase the risk of a fall as well, because they decrease alertness and cause drowsiness. Anti-depressants and drugs to treat high blood pressure may cause falls too, because they can cause a sudden drop in blood pressure and light-headedness or fainting in some people. Of course, too many alcoholic beverages can also result in a fall.

One-third of people aged 65 and over fall at least once a year, resulting in an injury severe enough to require a visit to the hospital. Since falls are such a common occurrence, my parents and I started a fall-prevention program around their home, which included improving interior and exterior lighting, removing clutter, protruding furniture, and electrical cords from high-traffic walkways, and replacing throw rugs with non-slip rubber-backed mats.

We also moved frequently used dishes, utensils, toiletries, and clothes to reachable shelves, where stretching, bending, and climbing could be avoided. Dad added a second handrail beside the stairs that went to the basement and installed a grab bar in the bathtub, the most slippery place in the house. Hardware stores and home health-care stores have many of the supplies and devices needed to prevent falls.

My parents decided it was time to change their footwear too, to increase their stability on their feet. They switched to rubber-soled shoes, slippers, and boots, and Mom threw out her flip-flops and backless slippers, as well as her high-heeled and sling-back shoes.

My father also hired someone to remove fallen leaves, and in the winter, snow and ice from the driveway and walkways. I spoke to him about the risk of a fall from climbing his ladder, so he reluctantly hired someone to paint the non-brick sections of their house.

Fall-Prevention Checklist for Around the House

Location	Elder-Proofing Initiatives
Kitchen	• Move frequently used dishes and utensils to easily reachable shelves • Add a non-slip mat in front of sink • Buy a stepstool with handrails
Bathroom	• Install grab bar on bathtub tiled wall and handrails on wall • Buy new rubber tub mat and bath mat • Put plastic transfer bench or chair in bathtub, if recovering from surgery • Install taller toilet or raised toilet seat, if needed • Install night light • Mount liquid-soap dispenser in bathtub or shower so seniors don't have to deal with slippery soap
Bedroom	• Install night light in bedroom and on the wall to the bathroom • Remove clutter from walkways
Living Room	• Remove throw rugs or put non-slip pads or mesh underneath • Remove electrical cords lying across floors • Eliminate clutter and protruding furniture from high-traffic areas
Stairs, Steps, Hallways, and Front & Back Entrances	• Improve lighting, and add overhead lights • Remove clutter • Add handrails to both sides of stairs • Put light switches at both top and bottom of stairs • Add rubber-backed mats • Add a chair for putting on shoes at one entrance

Footwear	• Ensure footwear has rubber soles • Throw out flip-flops as well as high-heeled, backless, and sling-back women's shoes and slippers
Outside	• Remove fallen leaves, snow, and ice from driveway and walkways

Seniors may also need to make some important lifestyle changes that involve becoming more physically active and improving their diet. Inactivity and lack of proper nutrition negatively affect bone health. Check with your parents' family doctor before starting any new exercise routine, but if he or she agrees that increasing physical activity is safe, then the earlier seniors start becoming active the better.

Weight-bearing and resistance exercises are best for building muscle and bone mass, as well as improving balance and coordination. Weight-bearing exercises, such as walking and dancing, use our feet and legs to work bones and muscles against the force of gravity. Resistance exercises, such as lifting weights, strengthen a particular muscle group, which in turn strengthens bones in that area. Strengthening thigh, core, or torso muscles, and the muscles that control ankles, take priority, since they are crucial to maintaining good balance.

Under the direction of a family doctor, a physiotherapist can develop a customized exercise program to accommodate a person's current medical conditions and physical limitations, and teach the senior proper exercise techniques to avoid injury. Tai chi, which focuses on slow, balanced movements, can also help to prevent falls. This ancient Chinese martial art is taught by the Taoist Tai Chi Society and YMCAs in many local communities.

Adopting a bone-healthy diet that includes calcium-rich foods, such as milk, cheese, and yogurt, will help to strengthen bones. When the calcium level in blood gets too low, our body steals it from our bones. Osteoporosis Canada recommends that adults over the age of 50 get 1,200 milligrams of calcium a day from all sources, and the best source is food. The organization's website (www.osteoporosis.ca) has a calcium calculator so seniors can calculate their daily calcium intake from foods. If they usually fall short, they should discuss the option of taking a calcium supplement with their family doctor.

According to Osteoporosis Canada, 800 to 2,000 international units (IU) of vitamin D a day is imperative, so that our bodies are able to absorb calcium. There are few food sources of vitamin D and sun is an unreliable source, so the organization recommends routine daily supplements for all Canadian adults year-round. Again, consult with your physician.

Caffeinated coffee, tea, energy drinks, and cola soft drinks increase the loss of calcium from the body through urine, so limit them to four five-ounce cups a day. Salt also increases urinary loss of calcium, so it should be limited to one teaspoon per day from all sources. Eating more fresh foods, and fewer packaged and fast foods with high salt content will help.

The senior's primary care physician should be involved in reducing the risk of a fall by conducting a falls-risk assessment, or giving a referral to a fall-prevention clinic. The investigation includes reassessing all medications and takes into account previous falls and fractures, sex, and age. Any changes in vision, balance, peripheral sensation, muscle strength, postural sway, and reaction time are also to be evaluated.

Falls can lead to fractures and the underlying cause of the fracture could be osteoporosis, which accounts for over 80 per cent of all fractures after age 50. It is, therefore, essential that the falls-risk assessment include a bone-mineral-density test. According to Osteoporosis Canada, "this bone disease leads to increased bone fragility and the risk of broken bones, particularly of the spine, hip, shoulder, and wrist." One in four women and at least one in eight men over the age of 50 has osteoporosis. The disease often goes undiagnosed, so you can see why this test is so critical.

If the assessment indicates that a senior has low bone density and is at high risk of falling, their doctor may prescribe a medication to slow down bone loss as well as refer them to a physiotherapist, to develop a regular exercise program that will safely increase bone mass as I described earlier. To further reduce the risk of falling, he or she may recommend that the patient be fitted for a walker or a cane. Make sure the cane has a rubber cap on the bottom to prevent slipping, and that a metal pick or cleat is added for outdoor walks in icy conditions.

As I learned, by their mid-30s, women start to lose 1 per cent of their bone mass each year. In the first five years following menopause, they can lose as much as 3 per cent a year due to much lower estrogen levels. I realized that if my mother had been tested for osteoporosis when she reached the age of 50, she could have been prescribed a medication during the most rapid period of bone loss. At that time, she should have been flagged as being at higher risk of developing osteoporosis, because being petite and weighing less than 60 kilograms (132 pounds), she had smaller bones than most women. For more information on osteoporosis and bone health, visit the Osteoporosis Canada website where you can sign up to receive their electronic newsletter, *COPING*.

Sarah Nixon-Jackle is a public health nurse and a member of the Saskatoon Falls Prevention Consortium. In the February 18, 2011, issue of *COPING*, she reported that the most common reasons people give for falling are, "I just wasn't paying attention," or "I thought I was still able to do . . . " She offered this advice that speaks to the need for all of us to adopt a more cautious approach to daily living: "Slow down and focus on one task at a time. Become more watchful of surroundings and anticipate risks. Be patient when trying to do a challenging task. Find a safe approach or ask for help."

I have a friend whose 88-year-old mother slipped in the middle of the night when she was getting off the toilet in her hospital room. She got wedged between the toilet and the wall and was there for more than four hours before someone found her. Fortunately, she wasn't injured, but the ordeal frightened her and her family. To reduce the risk of a fall and this type of distress, notify the charge nurse in a hospital or the director of care in a nursing home if your loved one is at high risk of falling. It is also important to find out what specific fall-prevention procedures are in place, and to ask that they be enforced for your parent or spouse.

These procedures commonly include having nursing staff assess at-risk patients when they are first admitted, by asking about their physical limitations, their normal sleeping patterns, and any mobility aids they use, such as a walker or a cane. Hospitals may also install bed and washroom alarms and bed siderails. An important element of hospital fall-prevention procedures is having nursing staff check on high-risk patients at regular intervals. Each nursing station decides on how often these patients are checked, depending on their current workload, but at a minimum it should be two to three times per eight-hour shift.

Reduce Risk of Adverse Drug Reactions

Seniors are more vulnerable than younger people to an adverse drug reaction, because they have a slower metabolism. A lower dose than the standard adult dosage may be safer and more effective. They are also more likely to have overmedication problems, because they tend to be taking more medications to control their increasing number of chronic ailments. These drugs may be prescribed, not just by their family doctor, but also by several medical specialists.

Seniors are more prone to medication mix-ups due to interactions with over-the-counter drugs or by not taking their medications as prescribed. These errors can lead to dizziness in older adults, causing them to fall. Sometimes, aging adults who show up in hospital emergency rooms with symptoms of life-threatening conditions could simply be suffering from overmedication, or from taking medications incorrectly.

Family-care leaders can help reduce the risk of adverse drug reactions by becoming knowledgeable about the medications that their loved one is taking. Start by preparing a list of every medication and the dosage levels. Then learn the reason for taking each medication, common side effects, and any potentially dangerous side effects. This list could be vitally important in a medical emergency.

Being on the lookout for dangerous side effects could save a life. When a senior has a poor reaction to a medication, notify the family doctor and pharmacist. Call 911 if he or she is showing life-threatening side effects, such as swelling of the tongue and mouth, difficulty breathing, a rapid heartbeat, a sudden drop in blood pressure or loss of consciousness.

Pharmacists can help by providing a list of all medications, potential side effects, and drug interactions. This service is often offered free of charge. Encouraging a senior to have all their medications filled at one pharmacy makes sense, so that the pharmacist can check for interactions each time a prescription is filled. It is also best to choose a pharmacy that provides a list of specific usage instructions for each prescription filled.

Encourage your loved ones to ask their family doctor, and any specialists they see, about the risks and benefits of a new medication. Discussing alternative medications and potential interactions with other prescribed drugs is also a good idea, before agreeing to take the prescription. By checking with their pharmacist too, they can further reduce the risk of a new medication altering or eliminating the effectiveness of the medications they are already taking. Don't forget to mention other over-the-counter medications, vitamins, or herbal supplements that they are taking.

Furthermore, before a senior is discharged from a hospital stay, ask a registered nurse assigned to them for a list of medications to stop taking and continue taking, and a list of new medications prescribed in the hospital. This medication reconciliation, which should also be sent to their family doctor, will help ensure their safety when they return home.

To reduce the risk of medication mix-ups, my mother purchased plastic daily-pill dispensers for her and my father. Her friend Sue came to visit once a week to fill their pill dispensers. That took the guesswork out of whether they had already taken their medications each day. Later on they arranged with their pharmacy to dispense their pills grouped together for each day in a monthly blister pack. This can certainly help seniors safely extend their independence.

When older adults are in a medical emergency situation in the hospital they are at greater risk of a serious drug complication, because they may need even more medications, and possibly an anaesthetic for surgery. When surgery is needed, seniors and their family-care leaders should ask their surgeon for a consultation with the anaesthesiologist who will be working with them. Families should enquire if there is a good option to a general anaesthetic for the particular surgery being done, one that may lower the risk of serious side effects, such as delirium and cognitive decline. A regional or local anaesthetic to suppress pain, combined with a medication to sedate patients, may be a better option than putting seniors in an unconscious state.

My mother and I had a meeting with her anaesthesiologist prior to oral surgery to remove infected roots from seven teeth. I had a chance to ask questions, and I learned that he planned to use neuroleptic anaesthesia, which would block her pain receptors without completely eliminating wakefulness. Her surgery went smoothly, she had no side effects from this type of anaesthesia, and she recovered fairly quickly.

Hospital-Acquired Infections

Older patients are much more likely than younger patients to contract infections and viruses in the hospital, because with age and age-related conditions, they have a weaker immune system. *Clostridium difficile*, also known as *C. difficile* (or *C. diff*) is one of the most common infections found in hospitals that can cause outbreaks among patients, and even death, especially among seniors. Symptoms may include watery diarrhea, fever, loss of appetite, nausea, and abdominal pain or tenderness.

People can become infected if they touch a contaminated hospital surface, such as a call button, a telephone, a bed siderail or table, a privacy curtain, or toilet, and then touch their mouth or nose. Health-care workers can spread the bacteria to other patients or contaminate surfaces through hand contact. This germ can even be found on stethoscopes and blood-pressure cuffs.

It takes courage, but family-care leaders should ask doctors and nurses to wash their hands before touching their sick loved one. All hospital visitors should do the same. Disinfecting the surfaces that their loved one and health-care professionals commonly touch in their hospital room will help reduce the risk of infection. A concentration of one part bleach to nine parts water should be high enough to kill this type of bacteria. Also, people who have a cold or the flu should refrain from visiting because patients likely have a weakened immune system, and viruses can more easily spread in such close quarters.

If a senior's surgery or other medical condition involves the use of a catheter to drain urine, family-care leaders should ask each day when it can be taken out. This inserted tube can increase the risk of developing a urinary tract infection, and should be removed as soon as it is no longer medically necessary. Family caregivers and other visitors can further reduce the risk of this type of infection by keeping their parent or spouse well hydrated, bringing them water to drink throughout the day.

Family caregivers also need to recognize the symptoms of a urinary tract infection in seniors, which are confusion, cloudy or bloody urine, strong or foul-smelling urine, or urine output that is much lower than fluids consumed. The urine consistency can be seen in the urine bag that is attached to the catheter and likely hanging by the hospital bed. If symptoms are present, notify the patient's nursing staff and request that the urine be tested for a possible infection as soon as possible. Catching a urinary tract infection early and treating it with a medication can help ensure a faster recovery.

There are a number of predictable medical crises that can be avoided. It doesn't take much effort to create a safer environment for aging family members, and there is a huge payoff. Seniors are likely to avert unnecessary suffering and stress that go hand-in-hand with a medical emergency. Avoiding a crisis can delay a downward spiral in health and extend a senior's independence. The reward for family members will be fewer fires to fight, and a delay in when they need to start their caregiving duties.

TOP TIPS

Extend Seniors' Independent Lives

- Eliminate the typical causes of the most common accidents that happen to seniors.
- Build a safety net that provides ready access to help when needed.

Creating Safer Home Environment Gives Peace of Mind

- Install a 24-hour-a-day personal emergency response system.
- Arrange for assistance from neighbours, friends, and family when seniors have questions or concerns, or are unable to handle problems on their own.
- Give house keys to trusted neighbours and family.

Help Prevent Falls

- Make house safer.
- Encourage seniors to adopt a bone-healthy diet and exercise program to increase muscle and bone mass and improve balance and coordination.
- Ask the family doctor to do a falls-risk assessment, test for low bone density, and treat to strengthen bone health, if necessary.

Help Prevent Adverse Drug Reactions

- Become knowledgeable about seniors' medications, and common and potentially dangerous side effects.
- Encourage seniors to have medications filled at one pharmacy, so with any new medication, a pharmacist can check for potential interactions.

- Buy a daily-pill dispenser to help avoid medication mix-ups.
- Explore alternatives to general anaesthetic for surgical procedures.

Help Prevent Hospital-Acquired Infections

- Fight off life-threatening C. *difficile* and other infections by disinfecting commonly touched surfaces in patient's room, and asking doctors, nurses, and visitors to wash their hands before touching your loved one.
- Reduce the risk of a urinary tract infection by asking nursing staff to remove catheter as soon as possible after surgery and keeping patient well hydrated.

Navigating the Health-Care Maze and Advocating for Mom

In the late afternoon on December 23, 2003, I was busy preparing for my mother's visit for the Christmas holidays when I was suddenly interrupted by the telephone. In an urgent-sounding voice, the administrator of my mother's retirement residence said, "Your mother has fallen and I think she might have broken her leg. An ambulance has just taken her to the hospital. I called Sue. She is on her way to meet your mother in the ER."

That call began a terrifying two-day ordeal because the hospital in Cobourg didn't have orthopaedic surgeons on staff. The attending physician called the nearest regional hospital, only to learn that there were seven orthopaedic emergencies ahead of Doris, so she was refused admittance. By the next morning, I was in a real panic waiting for our health-care system to find my mother a hospital with an available surgeon and a bed.

Because I realized there would probably only be skeleton operating-room staff on duty Christmas Day, I became my mother's tenacious advocate. I paged her family doctor and expressed my fear that if my mother didn't have surgery until December 26, she could die from a blood clot. In a stern voice, he said he was well aware of the problem and was waiting to hear back from a surgeon. In an attempt to raise his sense of urgency further, I told him that I was about to leave Toronto for Cobourg, and would drive to whichever hospital was going to perform my mother's surgery.

Mitch and I arrived at the hospital only to discover that Mom had just left. Within a few minutes, we were following her ambulance to the hospital in Belleville. When we arrived, Mom was relieved to see me and to have me take charge of the situation.

Within a half hour, we met her surgeon, who, after examining her X-ray, grumbled that he could drive a Mack Truck through the holes in her porous thigh bone. This was a telling sign of severe osteoporosis. He also complained that all the operating rooms were booked and he didn't expect to get Mom into surgery anytime before 11 p.m. Fearing that he might change his mind and bow out, I assured him that we would be there for the operation whenever it was. Mitch and I watched Christmas Eve turn into Christmas Day, and after two and a half hours my mother's surgery was complete. By 1:45 a.m. she had two plates and seven screws holding her brittle left femur bone in place.

Later that same week, Doris developed a blood clot in her leg, known as a deep vein thrombosis. It was a complication from surgery, despite having the operation performed within the critical first 48 hours. A blood-thinning medication was prescribed and all was well.

As a rookie family leader over the care and well-being of our mother, this medical emergency taught me how vital it is to get to know how the health-care system functions, especially in hospitals. I also realized that I needed to be better prepared for my advocacy role, because seniors are vulnerable to life-threatening medical emergencies requiring hospitalization and surgery, as well as a longer stay in a hospital.

They will eventually need an advocate when they are unable or too sick to speak for themselves, and when health problems are not being resolved quickly, or in a way that they would want, or in their best interest. As the chief advocate for Doris Inc., I learned a good deal about how to navigate the health-care system and become an effective advocate. My on-the-job training came from trial and error, lots of practice, and discussions with many health-care professionals.

A number of important aspects of navigating the health-care maze are covered in other chapters. For instance, how to find a good retirement residence is covered in chapter 9, the process to get into a nursing home is covered in chapter 8, and how to find a good nursing home is dealt with in chapter 10.

This chapter, however, focuses on explaining how the hospital health-care system operates, why elders need a family advocate, as well as how to become an effective advocate with family doctors, medical specialists, and administrators and nursing staff of seniors' residences and nursing homes.

HOW TO WORK BEST WITH HOSPITAL HEALTH-CARE PROFESSIONALS

Once a patient is admitted to the hospital, a health-care team is assigned to them based on the assessment of their medical conditions. The team could include many of the health-care professionals listed in the table below. They are the people who direct and provide care. A key member of this team is the attending physician, who is responsible for the overall care of patients assigned to him. He or she coordinates the diagnostic tests and treatments that are performed by medical specialists or surgeons.

The Typical Hospital Care Team

Care Team Member	Their Role
Triage Nurse (If visit starts in the ER)	• Interviews incoming patients to the emergency room • Makes decision on urgency of care needed, which determines how long a patient waits to see a doctor
ER Physician (If visit starts in the ER)	• Assesses and decides if patient will be admitted • May start tests and treatment, or call in specialists

(Continued)

Care Team Member	Their Role
Attending Physician	• Responsible for the care of a patient admitted to the hospital • Coordinates diagnostic tests, medical treatment, and care • Could be patient's family doctor, a surgeon, or other specialist with visiting privileges to the hospital; could also be a *hospitalist*, a family doctor assigned to a patient just while in the hospital
Medical Specialist and Surgeon	• Develops treatment plan, orders diagnostic tests and medications, and performs surgery or other treatments
Head Nurse and Charge Nurse	• Head nurse is in charge of a hospital ward, and usually works Monday to Friday, nine to five; at other times, the role is filled by a senior nurse known as a *charge nurse*. • Oversees nursing functions of a ward • Responsible for delivery of quality patient care
Nursing Staff	• Registered nurses carry out doctors' orders, assess and create nursing-care plans, and handle patients with more complex and unstable conditions • Registered or licensed practical nurses (RPN) monitor health status, carry out care plans, and administer medications and bedside nursing for stable patients • Personal support workers (PSW) provide assistance with activities of daily living, and assist RPNs and RNs
Discharge Planner (called a Social Worker in some hospitals)	• Called in if patient needs higher level of care when discharged than they had before hospital visit • Works with family and provincial community care agency to arrange for home care or a nursing-home placement
Pharmacist	• Monitors medications for side effects and interactions • Called in to find an alternative medication when patient is not responding to standard medications or dosages

Geriatric Clinic	• If patient has complex chronic diseases and newly arising issues they may be referred to a geriatric clinic or geriatrician
Dietitian	• Ensures any special dietary needs are met
Physiotherapist	• Helps patient with muscle/bone/joint rehabilitation
Occupational Therapist	• Helps patient overcome limitations and modify their home, so they can participate more fully in the activities of daily life

An ER nurse once told me that patients who come to a hospital emergency room often expect service on a first-come-first-served basis, like a fast-food restaurant. Hospitals operate on a priority, or *triage,* system that always treats the most critically ill patients first. Families need to learn to be patient, but they should contact the nursing staff if the waiting time seems excessive. In the ER, triage nurses assess patients' medical conditions using the Canadian Triage and Acuity Scale (CTAS), which classifies how urgently they need to be seen by an ER physician.

Canadian Triage and Acuity Scale[1]

Level	Priority Name	Condition Explanation	Condition Examples	Ideal Time
1	Resuscitative	Conditions that are threats to life or limb, or an imminent risk of deterioration	Cardiac/ respiratory arrest, major trauma, shock states, unconsciousness, severe respiratory distress	Immediately seen by doctor 98% of the time

(Continued)

[1] Source: *Canadian Journal of Emergency Medicine,* October 1999 and January 2008, and www.calgaryhealthregion.ca/policy/docs/1451/Admission_over-capacity_AppendixA.pdf.

Level	Priority Name	Condition Explanation	Condition Examples	Ideal Time
2	Emergent	Conditions that are a potential threat to life, limb, or function	Altered mental states, head injury, severe trauma, a heart attack, or a stroke	Within 15 minutes, 95% of the time
3	Urgent	Conditions that could potentially progress to a serious problem, requiring emergency intervention	Moderate trauma, asthma, gastrointestinal bleed, acute pain, acute psychosis, or suicidal thoughts	Within 30 minutes, 90% of the time
4	Less Urgent	Conditions related to patient age, distress, or potential for deterioration or complications	Headache, foreign body in eye, and chronic back pain	Within one hour, 85% of the time
5	Non-Urgent	Conditions that may be acute but non-urgent, or chronic with or without evidence of deterioration	Upper respiratory infection, sore throat, mild abdominal pain that is chronic or recurring	Within two hours, 80% of the time

An ER physician will usually see all patients classified as non-urgent, although they may have to wait for some time, if the ER is very busy with level 1–4 priorities. Non-urgent patients may be referred to other areas of the hospital or the health-care system, with or without being examined by an ER physician. This could happen, for example, if a family in crisis brings their elderly loved one to the ER because they don't feel they can care for them at home any longer. A social worker or discharge planner may be called in to explain the process to apply for a nursing-home placement, and then send them home.

Family-care leaders can bring the hospital health-care team up to speed on their loved one's medical issues when they are first admitted, by doing the following:

- Upon admission, immediately provide a list of the senior's medical history, current medications and dosages (including over-the-counter drugs and vitamins), current medical issues and symptoms, and any allergies.

- Bring all of the senior's medications to the hospital, so the ER physician can immediately see what medications he or she is taking, and so there won't be an interruption in the administration of medications.

- Bring the contact information for their family doctor and medical specialists.

- Bring a copy of the Power of Attorney for Personal Care document, if there is one.

Whether an elder's hospital visit starts in the emergency room or in the operating room, it is important for families to speak with one unified voice. They should provide the nursing staff with the contact information of one family member. Asking to be called at any time, day or night, if there has been a change in medical status will help keep family members informed and deeply involved in the elder's care.

When hospitalization is required for an elderly patient living with a number of chronic diseases, it is important for families to realize that the goal is often not to fix the problem, which usually isn't curable, but to address the acute phase of the related chronic condition, and to ease and control symptoms more effectively.

Health-care budgets, and therefore the availability of hospital nursing staff, will never be enough to meet all patients' needs. This is one of the realities of our public health-care system; however, families can help by pitching in when they visit their loved one, just as they would if they were sick at home. There are many ways that you can help.

Making patients feel as comfortable as possible, by helping them to eat, bringing them water to drink to keep them hydrated and so they can brush their teeth, finding an extra blanket if they are cold, and refreshing them by washing their face and hands will demonstrate your love, and your willingness to partner with the hospital care team. Asking nursing staff how you can help will always be a welcomed gesture.

Asking neighbours and friends or hiring caregiver-companions to visit and help your parent or spouse be as comfortable as possible in the hospital will give primary caregivers a much-needed break from their hospital duties.

Families should seek the assistance of the hospital discharge planner as soon as possible after their loved one has been admitted to the hospital, if returning home is not a safe option or if he or she lives alone and is likely to need support. This will get the senior plugged into the local community care agency early, and ensure your loved one receives the best discharge care plan once they leave the hospital.

If an elderly patient already lives in a nursing home, ask the discharge planner to assess whether the current nursing home has the capability of providing any specialized care that may be necessary. Asking if any temporary supports are needed and who can provide them is also a good idea.

Patients and their families need to know that they have the right to ask questions and raise concerns with any member of the health-care team. Ask questions about health status, diagnostic test results, and treatment options. Questions asked by family-care leaders are often based on their unique perspective and knowledge of the patient and their wishes, which can be very helpful to the health-care team.

Families can get their questions answered in a number of ways. An RPN assigned to a patient is a good person to ask about health status, medications, and turnaround times for test results. If they don't have the answers they should refer you to the RN. The head or charge nurse should be able to answer questions about the patient's care plan, diagnostic test results, and scheduled procedures. They will also be able to tell patients who their attending physician is, when they routinely visit the patient care ward, and how to reach him or her as well as other specialists.

Patients or their attorney for personal care have the right to see their active in-patient chart, which is a binder that includes the diagnosis, test results, treatment and nursing care plans, and vital signs. Families may need the help of a nursing staff member to interpret the data. This information will be harder to access once hospitals convert to electronic patient records. When that happens, patients or their substitute decision-maker will have to ask to look at this information on a hospital computer.

Once a person is discharged from a hospital, they can obtain their patient records, including test results, from their family doctor or the hospital's medical records department. Hospitals may charge a fee for this service, and because of the federal Privacy Act, a consent form must be completed to officially request the test results.

For information about the risks and benefits of treatment options, try to reach the attending physician, specialist, or surgeon while he or she is doing rounds. When having a conversation with an attending physician or specialist, it would be appropriate to ask how to best reach them with any further questions or concerns that might arise.

When families leave a message with the charge nurse for the patient's attending physician or specialist, they shouldn't assume that their message will go to the right person. Double-check after a few days, if a response is expected. If families have difficulty getting their questions answered, the discharge planner can arrange a family conference with the health-care team or a particular physician.

Occasionally, a family or patient may not have confidence in a specialist's recommended course of treatment, and when this happens, they have the right to ask for a second opinion. A list of physicians and specialists can be obtained from the website of the College of Physicians and Surgeons in each province, or by calling the local hospital medical staff officer.

WHY ELDERS NEED A FAMILY ADVOCATE

There are a number of reasons why elders often don't receive the medical attention they need to resolve all their many medical problems, unless they have a knowledgeable and involved advocate.

Elders Have More Chronic Diseases and Ailments

Elders may have several chronic diseases, such as heart disease, emphysema, diabetes, arthritis, or osteoporosis, which usually have a slow but steady downward progression. To make matters worse, the body's systems, such as circulation, immune, nervous, and digestion, deteriorate with age. Consequently, many elderly people require vigilant ongoing monitoring and management of their health care to avoid serious complications and a life-threatening acute incident, and to function as well as they can.

Elderly Patients Take Longer to Diagnose and Treat

Sometimes family doctors cannot address all of an elderly patient's many health problems during the same appointment, and must prioritize the order of health issues that they treat. For this reason, while a primary care physician can usually handle the routine medical problems of a young person in 10 minutes, it can take a half hour with a senior. Physicians are paid the same per appointment, so they are not compensated for the longer visits. They may, understandably, lose patience unless a family member is there to help make the call as efficient and productive as possible. Family-care leaders can help get the most out of the appointment by bringing a list of medical problems and symptoms, as well as questions and concerns. This will help reduce the length of the visit and ensure that the most important topics are covered.

Elderly People Tend to Play a Passive Role in their Health Care

Doris was typical of her generation. She let her family doctor lead while she played a passive role in her own health care, never questioning his decisions and advice. Sometimes though she would arrive home and realize she didn't understand what he asked her to do or why she was given a prescription. When a new medical issue arose she would rather wait than bother him, hoping that it would go away.

Many other elders have a similar attitude toward their health care and can be somewhat intimidated by authority figures. They may not be computer savvy, accustomed to doing their own medical research, or asking for advice from their family doctor before making medical decisions. If they have a number of ailments, they may not have much energy, which could make them even more passive when dealing with health-care professionals.

Disabilities May Hamper Good Communications

Many elders have some difficulty communicating with doctors and nurses because their hearing, eyesight, and memory may have gotten worse. They also reach a point where they can no longer drive and need to be driven to medical appointments.

Elders at Higher Risk of Adverse Consequences from Hospitalization

While hospitalized, older patients are more likely to have an adverse drug reaction, suffer from dehydration or bedsores, and contract viruses. They are also at a higher risk of complications and infections from surgical procedures.

They recover more slowly from surgical procedures and anaesthetic drugs can temporarily cause delirium, confusion, and agitation. When that happens, they may become uncooperative with health-care staff, which may interfere with their recovery. In patients with mild dementia, anaesthetics can accelerate cognitive decline, which is what happened to Doris after her leg surgery.

Older patients are also more likely to be misdiagnosed or to receive a treatment that doesn't work while they are in the hospital. Some diseases may be difficult to diagnosis because elders often exhibit different symptoms than younger people with the same disease. According to Dr. Barry Goldlist, director of geriatric medicine at the University of Toronto, "When they have heart disease, instead of experiencing shortness of breath, they may fall, or become incontinent or confused."[2]

Unfortunately, the functional abilities of elders may permanently decline after a hospitalization, leaving them less independent than they were before entering an acute care facility. With an understanding of the potential problems, family-care leaders should work with doctors and nurses to help reduce the risk of adverse consequences.

HOW TO BECOME AN EFFECTIVE ADVOCATE

I learned the skills of an effective advocate at a young age when my mother told me the story of how her father, Daniel Hillier, became the elected representative for the riding of Burin West in 1946. He was one of 45 delegates from across Newfoundland and Labrador who determined which constitutional choices Newfoundlanders should vote on in a referendum.

My grandfather was one of a small group of delegates, led by Joey Smallwood, who actively campaigned for confederation with Canada over three other options: remaining with a British-appointed government, becoming a British colony once again, and forming closer economic ties with the United States. Newfoundlanders voted to join confederation, and on April 1, 1949, Newfoundland and Labrador officially became the 10th province of Canada. From that moment on, Doris became as proud a Canadian as she was a proud Newfoundlander.

His example demonstrates that effective advocates get involved and care passionately about their cause, are persistent in their efforts, are respectful of different points of view, and communicate persuasively by raising justifiable points. These strategies can be applied to advocate effectively for an elderly patient in the following ways: by developing a good relationship with the health-care team, becoming well informed about medical problems and treatments, and searching for a better treatment when a senior's quality of life will suffer.

---

[2] Scott Anderson, "Care for the Aged," *University of Toronto Magazine*, Summer 2009.

Develop a Good Relationship with the Health-Care Team

The old adage that you can catch more flies with honey than vinegar is especially true when you want to resolve problems for your loved one that require increasing the sense of urgency, or changing attitudes or behaviours of health-care providers. A genuine smile and a pleasant demeanour just naturally make people want to be nice to you. Getting angry with health-care professionals is senseless. Emotional outbursts show disrespect, and may lead to resentment, and consciously or unconsciously getting back at you by treating your loved one poorly.

When I had a complaint about my mother's care, I always tried to communicate with physicians and nursing staff in a positive and constructive manner. I gained an appreciation for how hospitals, retirement residences, and nursing homes monitor and execute care for each person, and tried to understand the points of view of Mom's family doctor, surgeon, specialist, administrator, nurse, or personal support worker. That way, I could be much more realistic in my requests and suggested changes, and therefore increase the likelihood of a good outcome.

Being positive when your loved one isn't receiving the care that they need is much more difficult to accomplish in a life-threatening situation. However, the more you can act on what you know, rather than on your emotions, the more effective you will be. Try to raise justifiable concerns, not your feelings of stress and worry.

When dealing with the same health-care team over a period of time, get to know the staff, so you can communicate on a more personal basis. It is harder to turn down a request from someone you know. I enjoyed becoming part of the nursing-home community where my mother lived, and getting to know many of the people who worked there. I made it a priority to develop a good relationship with the administrator, director of care, and the nursing staff in the Alzheimer's unit, and to work as a team with them.

Regrettably, I did not make the same effort to get to know my parents' family doctor while they lived at home. My urgent call to him to find a hospital to fix my mother's broken leg might have gone better if I had. He might have also returned my phone call when Mom was first diagnosed with dementia. I learned from my mistake, however, and got to know and work better with her new doctor in the nursing home.

David and I adopted a tag-team approach to advocacy, whenever I uncovered concerns about Mom's health or her care in the nursing home. I discussed my concerns first with David and then openly with the nursing staff. When I was unable to solve problems at that level, my brother would call the administrator of the nursing home. They developed a very good working relationship and were always able to find a prompt solution that was in the best interest of both Mom and the nursing home.

Become Well Informed about Medical Problems and Treatments

Primary caregivers need to learn all they can about the medical history and current medical conditions of their loved one so that if their parent or spouse becomes incapacitated or has memory problems in the future, this knowledge could save their life.

I raised a warning flag when my mother developed an ulcer on one of her toes in her early 90s. Only I knew that the main arteries in my mother's legs had been 80 per cent blocked since she was in her early 70s. The nursing home's director of care responded by bringing in a wound-care specialist to help heal the ulcer, thus reducing the risk of gangrene.

Over the seven years that I looked after Mom, I tracked down and read information about Alzheimer's disease, osteoporosis, osteoarthritis, coronary heart disease, pacemakers, glaucoma, and intermittent claudication of the legs. This gave me a good understanding of Doris' many medical problems. I also learned about high-risk complications that needed to be prevented or managed carefully, such as circulatory problems, bedsores, and limb rigidity caused by immobility.

With knowledge, you will lower your stress level and gain confidence to ask health-care professionals questions about the care of your parent or spouse. That way, you will make the transition from being just a passive listener to being an active participant in discussions and decisions about treatment plans, and reasonable goals and expectations. The Internet is a fast and convenient tool that provides substantial depth and breadth of medical information; however, you need to know how to find websites that provide both accurate and current information.

Dr. Marla Shapiro, a Toronto physician, writer, and speaker, cautioned that while the Internet can be a very valuable tool, the quality of the information provided can be "variable, even inaccurate or wrong." In a November 7, 2006, article for the *Globe and Mail* entitled "Self-Diagnose off the Web at Your Peril," she recommended that Canadians "work with their physician to ensure the Internet is empowering and educating them in an appropriate way." Dr. Shapiro also provided the following tips from the U.S. Food and Drug Administration on how to best use the Internet to find medical information.

- Find out who runs the website and whether they are repu- table. That information should be readily available on the "About Us" section of the site.

- Is the website's purpose solely to inform, or is it to sell prod- ucts and/or raise funds? Remember, a claim that sounds too good to be true likely is not true.

- Information should be evidence-based and current. Reliable websites are reviewed and updated frequently.

- Look for the original source of the information. Sites that end in .gov are U.S.-government sponsored. University sites often end in .edu, and not-for-profit organizations usually use the extension .org.

Google is my favourite search engine, and I like Wikipedia (www.wikipedia.org) and WebMD (www.webmd.com) because they quickly get me up to speed on common diseases, are writ- ten in a language that is easy to understand, and are very user- friendly. When I need to go beyond basic health information I visit the trustworthy websites of disease charities, hospitals, especially the Mayo and Cleveland clinics, and government health sites, such as Health Canada (www.hc-sc.gc.ca).

Search for Better Treatment When Loved One's Quality of Life Will Suffer

David and I learned not to assume hospital staff, family doctors, and nursing homes will identify and resolve every problem that arises, or that they will always choose the best course of action. When a treatment was not working, we sought the advice of other experts and searched for a better option. Advocates should also consider asking for a referral to a geriatric clinic or a geriatrician when an elder has multiple chronic diseases and a family doctor or another specialist or surgeon is not making any progress. A geriatrician's in-depth knowledge of seniors may make all the difference in finding an effective treatment option.

I remember vividly a time soon after Doris moved into the nursing home when she went into a catatonic state and barely ate or kept her eyes open. My brother and I suspected that the painkiller she was taking was the culprit, because she had a similar reaction in the hospital, just after she broke her leg. With a great deal of apprehension, we overruled our mother's physician and the director of care by having her taken off a synthetic narcotic painkiller and switched to regular Tylenol.

I will never forget my visit to the nursing home a day after the switch in medications. As I rounded the corner and approached my mother's room, I heard her warm laugh and Newfoundland accent. Much to my relief, she had returned to her lively self.

We also asked our mother's doctor to take her off a drug used to reduce agitation and aggression in dementia patients, and a medication used to reduce anxiety. In both cases, we believed we made the wisest decisions for our mother. After searching for these drugs on the Internet, I learned (and had a doctor confirm) that these anti-psychotic drugs might increase the risk of a stroke or heart failure in elderly patients with dementia. As well, my mother didn't need the anti-anxiety drug that she had been taking because she was no longer in the emotional and behavioural instability stage of Alzheimer's disease.

Sometimes a proposed treatment, such as an amputation of a limb or appendage, will have a severe impact on quality of life. When there is time to explore other treatment options, good family advocacy and research can make a huge difference in the life of a parent or spouse.

A business associate of mine was able to save her mother from the painful and risky amputation of her feet, which had been recommended by two orthopaedic surgeons and a wound-care specialist. Her mother had diabetic ulcers on the balls of each foot that would not heal and there was a serious risk of gangrene. Through her own research on diabetic ulcers, she discovered that a treatment called topical pressurized oxygen therapy had success in healing ulcers.

My friend successfully appealed to the nursing home's director of care and the Ontario Ministry of Health and Long-Term Care for a special incubator to be brought into the facility. RNs, RPNs, caregivers, and my friend were all trained in how to administer the 90-minute treatment twice daily. Her mother was not permitted to walk during the therapy because of the risk of re-infecting her wounds. However, my friend's efforts and perseverance paid off because in five months the wounds healed. Her mother now walks unaided, and wears supportive shoes to prevent further ulcers.

Had her mother not had the benefit of this therapy she would have had her feet amputated, and been depressed and immobile for the rest of her life. Other residents in the same nursing home have since benefited from this treatment with equally impressive results. My friend is a good example of an effective family advocate who embodies my grandfather's strong advocacy skills of passion, determination, and diplomacy.

When an elder suffers from a broken hip or leg, or from a stroke, they often remain warehoused in a hospital for far too long, without receiving intensive rehabilitation. Their loss of mobility often leaves them worse off by the time they are finally discharged. My mother spent three months in the hospital when she broke her femur bone. By March 2003, she could still not put any weight on her left leg because it hadn't completely healed, so, very sadly, I purchased a wheelchair for her.

During most of this time, Doris required complex continuing care, but no longer needed the intensity of resources and services provided by an acute-care hospital. She was therefore designated by her attending physician as a hospital resident needing an alternate level of care (ALC), because the retirement residence where she lived did not offer the higher level of care that she needed. She spent so much time in the hospital only because she was waiting for a nursing-home placement.

To handle my mother's rehab, I unwisely relied upon brief physiotherapy sessions three to four times a week, arranged through the hospital and nursing home. My mother didn't have the mental capability to stretch and do physiotherapy exercises on her own, so she received very limited benefit from their efforts. Doris' legs became permanently bent at the knees from sitting all day in a wheelchair. The image of my mother sleeping with two pillows tucked beneath her knees, in order to relax her tight and shortened hamstring muscles, haunts me to this day.

I have since learned that I should have advocated for an integrated restorative program for my mother, going from an acute-care hospital to a rehabilitation hospital and then to a nursing home, or wherever she lived at that time. A stay in a rehabilitation hospital with intensive therapy six days a week for three weeks, once she was stable after surgery, might have significantly improved her outcome. Before being discharged, she would have been reassessed and specific direction provided for continued intensive therapy, once she was placed in a nursing home.

Stroke victims and seniors with hip fractures, with or without dementia, can also benefit from the same integrated restorative program. In October 2010 the South East Ontario Local Health Integration Network announced a new initiative to design a more integrated restorative treatment and care program. This approach will hopefully become a reality across the country in the future. In the meantime, advocates should lobby for this integrated treatment plan, including a stay in a rehabilitation hospital.

Looking back, my brother and I both realize that by working closely and collaboratively with the people in Mom's health-care teams, and by advocating to resolve her health problems, we made a huge difference in her quality of life. On our watch, Doris received surgery to mend her broken leg, laser eye surgery to prevent blindness caused by glaucoma, and surgery to remove infected roots of teeth, so she could eat well again. We got her taken off medications when she had a dangerous reaction, when there was a risk of harmful side effects, and when she no longer needed them. As well, we prevented serious bedsore problems that can surface with immobility.

It is important to get involved and do the best you can for your parent or spouse when they need you to look out for their best interests with health-care providers. Of course, you will make some mistakes, but you will learn from them and find new ways to avoid problems, make better decisions, and improve your loved one's quality of life.

TOP TIPS

Elders Will Eventually Need an Advocate

- Elders require an advocate when they are unable or too sick to speak for themselves, and when their health problems are not being resolved.

Get Involved in Your Elder's Care

- Elders receive better care when their family gets involved and works collaboratively with their health-care teams.

Learn How Hospitals Operate

- A health-care team is assigned to each patient.

(Continued)

- An attending physician coordinates all the care of patients assigned to him.
- Discharge planners will set the wheels in motion to arrange for home care or a nursing-home placement, if needed.

Learn Patients' Rights

- Patients and the person(s) appointed under their Power of Attorney for Personal Care have the right to:
  - ○ ask questions, and should ask questions, based on their own unique perspective and knowledge of medical history and wishes
  - ○ ask for a second opinion, if they do not have confidence in a specialist's recommended treatment plan
  - ○ see their active in-patient hospital chart that contains their diagnosis, test results, treatment and care plan, and vital signs

A Geriatrician and a Rehabilitation Hospital Can Be a Godsend

- A geriatrician may be able to find an effective treatment option when an elder has multiple chronic diseases, and when other doctors are not making progress.
- Stroke victims and elders with broken legs and hips can benefit from intensive restorative therapy provided by a rehabilitation hospital.

Knowledgeable Advocates Make Better Care Decisions

- Learn about your elder's historical and current medical conditions and treatments.

- Learn about high-risk complications that need to be prevented or managed.

Develop a Good Relationship with the Health-Care Team

- Get to know the health-care team so you can communicate on a more personal basis. It is harder to turn down a request from someone you know.

Be Persistent

- Keep trying to reach doctors to ask your questions and raise concerns. The squeaky wheel gets the grease.
- Keep searching for a better option when a recommended treatment will dramatically lower your loved one's quality of life.

Advocates Can Accomplish More with Honey than Vinegar

- A genuine smile and a pleasant demeanour make people want to be nice to you.
- Communicate in a constructive and respectful manner.
- Make realistic requests, based on an understanding of the other's point of view.
- Try to raise justifiable concerns, not your feelings of stress and worry.

8

Choosing the Right Type of Living Arrangements

When my father died, the light of my mother's life flickered out and her world would never be as bright again. Her friend, Pauline, dropped in on her unexpectedly one late afternoon in November 2002, and found her sobbing quietly in her living room, in the dark. Doris came from a large and very loving family of eight and she had been married to Ed for 55 years, so living alone proved to be unbearable for her.

Her dementia symptoms were much more pronounced at about this time, too, and my brother and I both realized that Mom could no longer look after her house or herself safely on her own. If she was to live as independently as possible, she definitely needed full-time support. Mom, David, and I considered various living arrangements and decided that a retirement residence, where she could make new friends and participate in recreational activities, would be the best option.

David and I felt very guilty that we did not offer our mother the option of moving in with either one of us; however, as two middle-aged adults in promising relationships and with busy work and travel schedules, we felt that we wouldn't be able to give her the attention she deserved. Since Mom used a walker, our homes presented too many obstacles, such as stairs and sloped driveways to climb. We would also be taking her away from her comforts, good friends, neighbours, doctor, and church that were nearby in Cobourg.

The word *home* takes on greater meaning as we age, evoking feelings of comfort and security and memories of happy times with family, neighbours, and friends. Losing a home is another great loss in life for someone newly widowed. Most seniors detest change of any kind, and the more they feel they are losing control the more they fight to hang on to their independence. Men may be more reluctant to make living arrangement changes than women, because many of them are used to running their own show, and may have higher needs for independence and privacy.

In a medical crisis, seniors may be in denial of the long-term effects of their medical condition, believing that they will be back to their old selves in no time. Unfortunately, there are often physical restrictions, and for some, cognitive impairment that reduce their ability to live independently.

When a spouse or adult child sees that their loved one is struggling and his or her care needs have increased, they should take on a leadership role over the decision-making process to ensure that their loved one gets into the right place at the right time, where their needs for a higher level of care will be met, and where their safety can be assured. If a senior is deemed mentally capable, however, they cannot be placed in a retirement residence or nursing home against their wishes. Consent to admission into a nursing home is a stipulation of provincial governments' long-term care legislation. Ultimately, seniors have the legal right to live at their own risk.

Dignity and self-determination are valued by everyone, regardless of age. When a person has spent most of their life looking after themselves and others, it may feel disrespectful to have the very person whom they've raised suddenly tell *them* what to do. Discuss your love one's fears and concerns, talk respectfully about their health issues and the impact they will have, then negotiate the living arrangements. Navigating change isn't easy.

If your aging parent insists that he or she will never leave their home, consider contacting your provincial community care agency or hiring an eldercare consulting firm, both of which can offer advice, support, and information about living arrangement options. As objective third-parties, these geriatrics experts may be able to help your loved one reconsider lifestyle changes.

With time, reason usually prevails, and a senior agrees to a change in living arrangements. However, if a senior with dementia has reached a stage where their ability to reason and make sound decisions is impaired, then it would be appropriate to have their mental competency assessed, which their primary care physician can arrange. If they are deemed mentally incompetent, then their substitute decision-maker for personal care can make living arrangement decisions that are in the senior's best interest.

Once a decision to change living arrangements has been made, the next critical step is to select the best accommodations option, such as staying at home with help, moving in with family, or moving into some kind of seniors' residence. The following table lists the living arrangements that are commonly used for each stage of decline: supportive living, assisted living, dependent living, and palliative care, as explained in chapter 4 on page 62.

Accommodations Options for Each Stage of Decline

Accommodations Options Commonly Used	Stage of Decline			
	Supportive Living	Assisted Living	Dependent Living	Palliative Care
1. Stay at home with help	✓	✓		
2. Move in with family	✓	✓	✓	
3. Seniors' supportive housing	✓			
4. Retirement residence	✓	✓		
5. Retirement condominium	✓			
6. Life-lease apartment	✓			

(Continued)

Accommodations Options Commonly Used	Stage of Decline			
	Supportive Living	Assisted Living	Dependent Living	Palliative Care
7. Continuing-care retirement community	✓	✓	✓	✓
8. Nursing home			✓	✓

The living arrangements that seniors and their families choose are only the right choice if they include the right level of care each time seniors' care needs increase. Seniors and their families shouldn't be swayed by marketing brochures, magazines, websites, or sales pitches. Selling approaches usually capitalize on our dream of living a carefree, active, and healthy life until the day we die. Details about the level of care provided, and the availability and professionalism of staff are often scanty, buried in text, or not provided at all. Maintaining a high quality of life is, of course, extremely important, but if a loved one doesn't receive the care they need, then he or she will suffer.

Apart from acute hospital care and rehabilitation after an accident, a stroke, or surgery, there is an increasing level of care that will likely be needed by seniors as they transition through some or all of the stages of decline. Finding the answers to the following three questions will help aging seniors and their family choose the right level of care and type of living arrangements:

1. For each stage of decline, what level of care is needed and what living arrangement options can provide that care?
2. What are the real cost differences between living arrangement options?
3. Which living arrangement option is best?

SUPPORTIVE-LIVING STAGE

A description of the care needed and most commonly used living arrangement options for the supportive-living stage are provided next.

Care Needed

Care at the supportive-living stage should provide some or all meals and snacks, weekly laundry and housekeeping, and a responsible person to be available 24-hours a day, or a personal medical alert monitoring system, in case of an emergency. It should also include help with obtaining and taking medications, and a minimal to moderate level of assistance with self-care, such as bathing, if needed.

Accommodations Options

Stay at Home with Help

Independent seniors can choose to live in their own house, buy an adult-only condominium, or rent a suite in a seniors' apartment building, in order to eliminate outside chores and to be with people with similar interests. In any of these situations, volunteer or hired help can provide supportive-living care, and a personal medical alert system can be installed.

Seniors' Supportive Housing

Seniors' supportive housing is non-profit housing run by municipal governments or non-profit organizations, such as faith or cultural groups. This option offers people with modest incomes a low-rent option, or for those who qualify, government-subsidized rent, so they pay no more than 30 per cent of their monthly income. Rents are likely to range from $600 to $1,200 per month, but will vary across the country. Seniors must apply for supportive housing through their provincial community care agency.

Singles and couples can rent mostly fully equipped bachelor, or one- or two-bedroom apartments. There may be a waiting list for the most popular apartment buildings. This alternative provides homemaking and a minimal to moderate level of personal care. The actual level of support will vary. Care services may be provided by on- or off-site services, and there may or may not be a staff member available in the evenings and overnight, if there is an emergency.

Retirement Residences

Retirement residences are operated mostly by private corporations that charge a monthly rent for accommodations and a fee for meals and care services. Provincial governments do not subsidize rents. According to Derek Mercey, publisher of *The Care Guide,* there are three retirement-residence formats in Canada that provide increasing levels of care: independent supportive living, retirement care, and assisted living.

The independent supportive-living retirement format offers condo-style apartments to seniors who are still healthy and active. Housekeeping and laundry services are provided, and singles and couples can cook their own meals in their kitchen, or opt for the convenience of eating some or all of their meals in a common dining room. No hands-on personal care assistance is usually available, however, so this format is inappropriate for the supportive-living stage. Monthly rents for a private apartment for one person range from $2,000 to $5,000, depending on the area, size of apartment, and the extent of amenities offered.

The retirement-care format is designed for seniors who need supportive-living care. Mom moved into this type of residence, which met her care needs until she could no longer walk and developed significant cognitive impairment. It provides three meals a day, weekly housekeeping and laundry, 24-hour supervision, an emergency call-bell system in bedrooms and bathrooms, administration of medications, and a minimal to moderate level of assistance with personal care, such as help bathing.

Apartments tend to be smaller than the independent supportive-living retirement format, although there may be a kitchenette. Monthly rents for a private apartment for one person range from $2,000 to $6,000, depending on the area, size of apartment, and the extent of care services and amenities offered. Monthly rents for a semi-private room with a shared washroom, if available, may be as low as $1,500.

Retirement Condominium

Retirement condominiums offer seniors an ownership option. They are attached or linked to a retirement residence and offer condo residents meals and amenities for a monthly fee, and housekeeping, personal care, and health services on an à-la-carte fee basis.

Life-Lease Apartment

A life-lease is a housing arrangement, mostly offered by a non-profit or charitable organization, in which seniors purchase the right to occupy their apartment and use the common area amenities. Residents do not purchase their condo-style apartment, just the right to occupy it. The price can vary greatly, from $30,000 to $300,000, depending on the real-estate market and the cost of building the condo-style facility. When seniors leave, they sell their right and receive market value at the time of sale; however, if there is a buy-back clause, residents receive a specified guaranteed price when they leave.

Residents also pay a monthly occupancy fee that covers their share of the building operating costs and normal apartment costs, such as taxes, insurance, and utilities, depending on the size of the apartment. These fees can be as low as $250 a month, but may be higher in some areas. Residents typically have access to some or all of the services of a retirement-care model of retirement residence, for additional costs.

Continuing-Care Retirement Community

Continuing-care retirement communities give residents the option of "aging in place" and having the continuity of working with the same management team. They usually include independent-lifestyle suites in one area, assisted-living apartments in another area, and a nursing home. Seniors can settle in these communities as a couple or on their own while still independent. When needed, one or both of them can move to a unit with a greater level of care with little disruption of their life. The one caveat is that they need to be placed on a nursing-home waiting list as soon as they reach the dependent-living stage, so that hopefully they can obtain a nursing-home placement in the same complex. If they can do that, they will be able to stay in the same community from independent living until they die.

This continuing-care model reduces the stress on family caregivers who have to find new accommodations each time their loved one goes beyond the care capabilities of their existing residence. Unfortunately, there are only about 200 of these seniors' communities available across Canada. However, according to Nancy Solomon, director of communications at the Ontario Retirement Communities Association (ORCA), "Investors are seriously looking at this model for the future of retirement living."[1]

ASSISTED-LIVING STAGE

A description of the increased care needs and three most commonly used living arrangement options for the assisted-living stage are provided below.

Care Needed

Care at the assisted-living stage should provide all meals, and weekly laundry and housekeeping. Most people need round-the-clock supervision, ideally provided by a registered or licensed practical nurse, or at least by a responsible person in a home environment. A call-bell monitoring system should be available in bedrooms and bathrooms. Toward the end of the early stage of Alzheimer's disease, a senior often needs an assisted-living level of care.

Assisted-living care also involves the administration of medications, which includes monitoring their effectiveness. A moderate level of assistance with personal care should also be provided, such as bathing, dressing, getting up from chairs, and being escorted when walking, if needed. Depending on the complexity

---

[1] Nancy Solomon, telephone interview, September 2010.

of illnesses, monitoring of vital signs by a registered nurse may be required. There may also be a need for physiotherapy and occupational therapy, so that residents can participate more fully in activities of everyday life.

Accommodations Options

Stay at Home with Help

When a senior reaches the assisted-living stage, his or her spouse or children will need to arrange for help with household chores and maintenance. Live-in caregivers, government-funded home care and/or nursing and personal care services should be considered to augment the care provided by the family.

Move in with Family

The family may offer to move their frail parent in with them, if they have the ability to provide an assisted-living level of care in their own home. They can handle the administration of medications under the direction of the senior's family doctor. If the primary caregiver works outside the home, he or she will need to arrange for companionship, nursing and personal care, and respite so they can take a break.

Retirement Residences

Assisted-living retirement residences, also known as care or rest homes in some provinces, are designed for individuals at the assisted-living stage. They may or may not have a registered nurse on staff, so it is important to ask. Medications should be administered by a registered or licensed practical nurse. Personal support workers and health-care aides are not trained or certified in medication administration. Some of these facilities have a secure "memory care" wing, customized for people with an early stage of dementia, where they can wander freely, but cannot leave.

Assisted-living facilities can be in a stand-alone building, or a separate wing or floor of a retirement residence that also offers the independent-supportive or retirement-care format. In the latter two cases, residents are charged for assisted-living care services on an à-la-carte fee basis.

Monthly rents for a private apartment for one person can vary from $3,500 to $6,000, depending on the size of apartment, and on the amenities and care services provided. Some facilities offer shared and semi-private apartments that carry a monthly rent ranging from $2,600 to $3,000.

DEPENDENT-LIVING CARE STAGE

A description of the more complex care needs and the two most commonly used living arrangement options for the dependent-living stage are provided below.

Care Needed

Dependent-living care augments the supportive- and assisted-living care services with an increased level of medical intervention, as illnesses become more disabling and life threatening. A registered nurse and an on-call attending physician should regularly monitor residents' medical conditions. Supervision is usually required to reduce the risk of falling, as seniors become feeble and less stable on their feet. As eating becomes more difficult, dietitians are necessary to ensure proper nutrition.

Medications should be administered to seniors and round-the-clock assistance is usually needed with most activities of daily life, such as dressing, eating, using the toilet, hygiene, dental care, and mobility. Physiotherapy is often needed to ease the joint and muscle pain associated with immobility and osteoarthritis. Foot care, provided by a registered nurse every six weeks, is often needed to cut toenails, and to help prevent ingrown toenails, calloused skin, and fungus from growing underneath toenails.

Seniors who have reached the middle stage of Alzheimer's disease usually need dependent-living care provided by specially trained nursing personnel. They will function best in a secure area where they are free to wander, and in an environment designed to stimulate them mentally.

Accommodations Options

Live with Family

A family may decide to continue caring for a frail parent or spouse in their home despite their having reached the dependent-living stage. This option will likely require a significant time commitment from the family and could become very costly.

A visiting registered nurse will need to monitor their care, and personal support workers may also be needed to help the primary caregiver and offer respite. These services may be partially covered by government-funded home care; hiring care staff privately or through an agency is also an option. Family caregivers can administer medications themselves with a doctor's supervision.

Nursing Homes

Long-term care homes, commonly referred to as nursing homes, homes for the aged, or long-term care facilities, take care of residents who have reached the dependent-living stage of decline. Nursing homes are owned and operated mostly by private corporations, but also by municipal governments and non-profit corporations, such as faith, community, ethnic, or cultural groups.

Nursing homes provide dependent-living care in a secure setting, including medical supervision by a registered nurse 24 hours a day. Registered or licensed practical nurses, who are one level below registered nurses, provide medication management and medical care. They also supervise personal support workers or health-care aides, who provide residents with whatever personal care they need on a 24-hour-a-day basis.

Residents also have access to an on-call physician, a dietitian, and a physiotherapist. Meals, laundry, and a daily cleaning service are also provided. Most, but not all, nursing homes have a separate secure wing for seniors with dementia.

Provincial governments set the monthly fees that nursing homes charge residents. The Ontario government pays for the nursing-care portion of costs and residents pay for their accommodations and meals. In 2010–11, monthly fees in Ontario were $1,620 for basic accommodations, which have two to four residents to a room. A semi-private room with a shared washroom cost $1,863, and a private room cost $2,167.

No one will be refused admission to a nursing home if they do not have the financial means to pay their monthly fee, as long as they have a valid provincial health card. A subsidy that will reduce their fee is available on basic accommodations only.

PALLIATIVE-CARE STAGE

A description of the very specialized care needed and the three living arrangement options available for the palliative-care stage are provided below.

Care Needed

Once a senior becomes terminally ill, he or she usually needs hospice palliative care. This often involves 24-hour assistance with personal care, monitoring of vital signs and assessment of medical needs by a registered nurse, and ordering of needed medications by an on-call attending physician. Loved ones typically need pain management and physical comfort as their body starts to shut down. They often also have emotional and spiritual needs in their final months, days, or hours of life that can be met by family members, caregiver-companions, pastoral care visitors, and hospice volunteers.

Accommodations Options

Live with Family

At the palliative-care stage, family members may decide to bring their loved one home from the hospital to die. If they do, they will likely need to arrange for nursing supervision and personal care, some of which may be covered by provincially funded home care. They should also consider arranging for hospice care and pastoral care volunteers to visit to make their loved one more comfortable in their final days, and to provide respite for the primary caregiver.

Nursing Homes

Nursing-home residents who reach the end of their life can benefit from the palliative care provided by the nursing staff, who have grown to know them well and understand their individual care needs. Family caregivers should consider arranging for hospice volunteers to visit in the nursing home, unless they already have caregiver-companions visiting on a regular basis. Pastoral care visitors should also be considered.

Palliative-Care Unit in a Hospital

If a hospital has a palliative-care unit and a bed is available, this is a far better place to die than in a regular acute-care hospital ward, where the focus is on saving lives. The palliative-care team manages pain and symptoms, as well as providing psychological, social, and spiritual support. Hospitals, however, can be a very frightening place for people with dementia, so nursing homes are a more reassuring place for them to die.

BENEFITS OF MAKING THE RIGHT CHOICES

Getting elders in the right place, with the proper level of care at the appropriate time improves their well-being, and reduces the stress level of their primary caregivers. I know a kind gentleman who couldn't bear the thought of putting his wife in a nursing home, so she lived in a very beautiful memory wing of an assisted-living retirement residence for far too long.

He assumed that the care she received was sufficient for her needs, and it was, until she reached the middle stage of Alzheimer's disease, and needed dependent-living care.

Eventually, she got into a nursing home, where she quickly gained much-needed weight, and benefited from nursing supervision and personal care 24 hours a day, an on-call physician, a dietitian, and more appropriate bathing facilities.

REAL COST DIFFERENCES BETWEEN ACCOMMODATIONS OPTIONS

Cost is often one of the most important factors when deciding between different living arrangement options. An *apples* to *apples* cost comparison that identifies the *real* cost differences between options can help families choose the right type of living arrangements at the right time.

At the supportive-living stage, families often compare the cost of living at home with hired help to the cost of living in a retirement residence, where supportive care is provided. At the assisted- and dependent-living stages the cost comparison is usually between moving in with a family member, and an assisted-living retirement residence or a nursing home. Either way, the cost comparison between the home and a seniors' residence should include only the costs that will be different between the two options, such as the roof over their head, care, and food. The comparison should exclude common expenses that will be incurred regardless of where a senior lives, such as clothes, personal care products, and spending money.

Living at Home with Help versus a Retirement Residence in the Supportive-Living Stage

Seniors usually think it is far less expensive to live in their own house than in a retirement residence; however, they often overlook some of their house expenses, and the extra cost of hiring services to maintain their independence, such as lawn cutting, snow removal, and house cleaning. The biggest area of oversight is an opportunity cost, meaning the income lost from living in a house that could be sold and the money invested to earn income to pay for eldercare. The actual cost differences aren't usually as great as they first appear. The table below shows a cost comparison for a woman who lives alone in a mortgage-free house, with net equity of $250,000, in Kitchener-Waterloo, Ontario. Her annual house expenses are estimated at $12,000, and her supportive-living expenses at $4,000.

Living at Home with Help versus a Retirement Residence

Living at Home with Help		Retirement Residence
House & Food Expenses	Cost/Year	Cost/Year
Property taxes	$3,000	Retirement-Care Format
Utilities	3,800	in Kitchener/Waterloo
Insurance	1,000	
Repairs and maintenance	1,200	
Food	3,000	
Total House & Food Expenses	**$12,000**	
Supportive-Living Expenses		
Lawn care and snow removal	1,300	
Laundry and housekeeping services	2,000	
Medical alert monitoring 24 hours/day	700	
Total Supportive-Living Expenses	**$4,000**	
Opportunity Cost	7,500	
Total Annual Costs	$23,500	$26,400–$31,200

The next step is to calculate the opportunity cost of staying in the house. It is calculated by multiplying the net equity in the home by an estimated rate of investment return. I have used a 4 per cent investment return in my example, which would generate $10,000 in income each year. After taxes, the net income generated would be approximately $7,500, or 3 per cent of the $250,000. Therefore, her total cost of staying in her home would be $23,500. If the house value were higher, then the opportunity cost, and therefore her cost of staying in the home, would be even higher.

By comparison, her rental costs for a retirement-care model of retirement residence in Kitchener-Waterloo are estimated to be between $26,400 and $31,200 annually. Since this option is almost as cost-efficient as living at home, her decision should be based on her personal preference. This cost comparison example illustrates the type of cost analysis that should be done at the supportive-living stage of decline.

Moving in with Family versus an Assisted-Living Residence

Family caregivers usually think it is considerably less expensive for them to provide care for a parent or spouse in their own home, than to have them move into an assisted-living retirement residence. This depends on how much care is needed. They may lose sight of all the work that is involved in an assisted-living level of care, the special nursing skills that may be required, and the time it all takes.

If a primary caregiver cannot do everything, then someone else must, and some tasks may be better handled by hired professionals or through community home care. If a primary caregiver is determined to handle all the tasks by herself or himself, then they may not have a life of their own, and their loved one may not receive the quality care that he or she requires.

Every family's financial situation, support system, living arrangements, and health issues are very different. Despite these variables, the cost-comparison example that follows illustrates the type of analysis that should be done at the assisted-living stage of decline. This scenario assumes a daughter, who works 20 hours a week outside the home, has no backup family support, and hires nursing help to care for her father in her home. He has amyotrophic lateral sclerosis (ALS) and needs help with dressing, hygiene care, and mobility. His balance is poor, so he can't be left alone because of the risk of falling. The care costs in the table assume that caregiver-companions, such as the ones I hired for my mother, are hired privately, but the costs of personal support workers and registered nurses are hired through a home-care agency, such as Victorian Order of Nurses.

Moving In with Family versus an Assisted-Living Residence

Living with Family Caregiver				Assisted-Living Residence
Assisted-Living Care	Cost Rate	Cost Assumptions	Cost/Year	Cost/Year
Respite stay for elder in a nursing home	$35/day	2 weeks/year	$500	Small Semi-Private Apartment, $36,000, if available
Caregiver-companions	$18/hour	35 hours/week, 50 weeks/year	31,500	
Personal support worker	$28/hour	4 hours/week, 50 weeks/year	**5,600	Small Private Apartment, $42,000
Registered nurse	$60/hour	4 hours/month	**3,000	Large Private Apartment, $60,000
Total Care Costs			**$40,600**	
Less Gov't. Home Care			**8,600	Large Apartment with Kitchenette, up to $72,000
Net Care Costs			32,000	
Food Costs			2,000	
Total Annual Costs			**$34,000**	

If a case manager with the provincial community care agency assessed her father's home-care needs and then hired and paid for four hours per week of personal-support-worker time and four hours a month of registered-nurse time, then the cost of care would be reduced from $40,600 to $32,000. The total cost of care and food would then be $34,000, rather than $42,600.

In this scenario, it would be as cost-efficient for the father to live in a small apartment in an assisted-living retirement residence, as it would be for him to live with his daughter. The toll on the daughter of providing care, while still working, and having little time for herself is a huge cost, although not quantifiable, that should be considered in the cost comparison.

Live with Family versus a Nursing Home in the Dependent-Living and Palliative-Care Stages

At the dependent-living and palliative-care stages, the at-home model of providing dedicated supervision, nursing, and personal care to only one person is typically far more expensive than the nursing-home model of providing shared care to a group of residents.

There are so many variables involved at these stages that it is hard to predict what any one person will need in nursing and personal care. However, the chart below estimates that if 24-hour-a-day nursing and personal care are required, then $84,400 is the least it will cost, if care is provided totally by outside services, with the maximum coverage by provincial government-funded home care.

Live with Family versus a Nursing Home

Living with Family Caregiver				Nursing Home
Dependent-Living Care	Cost Rate	Cost Assumptions	Cost/Year	Cost/Year
Respite stay for elder in a nursing home	$35/ day	2 weeks/year	$500	Ontario, mid-2010 to mid-2011

Caregiver-companions	$18/ hour	13 hours/ day, 50 weeks/ year	81,900	Basic Accommodations, $19,440 Semi-Private, $22,356 Private Room, $26,004
Personal support worker	$28/ hour	3 hours/day, 50 weeks/ year	**29,400	
Registered practical nurse	$38/ hour	7 hours/day, 50 weeks/ year	**93,100	
Registered nurse	$60/ hour	1 hour/day, 50 weeks/ year	**21,000	
Total Care Costs			**$225,900**	
Less Maximum Gov't. Home-Care Coverage			**143,500	
Net Care Costs			82,400	
Food Costs			2,000	
Total Annual Costs			**$84,400**	

Every provincial community care agency covers a different amount of home care, and the support varies from year to year, depending on budget allocations. In Ontario in 2010, the maximum coverage was 3 hours a day of personal care and 8 hours a day of nursing care. If provincial government-funded home care covers a maximum of 11 hours a day for palliative care, then family caregivers or hired caregiver-companions need to cover the other 13 hours in a day. For the dependent-living stage, when a senior's condition is considered stable, home-care coverage would likely be considerably less than the 11 hours a day of maximum coverage.

Compared to this example, the cost of care for your loved one who lives with you will be *lower* by the extent that you provide care without any help, and by the number of hours of needed care that is less than 24. The cost of care will be *higher* by the extent that the community care agency provides fewer than 11 hours of care coverage.

Often overlooked are the costs of home modifications to maximize independence, and address the safety and mobility needs of a disabled parent or spouse. These costs can be considerable when a ramp or lift needs to be installed to accommodate a wheelchair, a second handrail is required on all steps, or specialized bed and bathroom aids are required. The list of modifications and gadgets can go on and on. The bottom line is: nursing-home costs are usually far lower than the cost of providing dependent-living and palliative-care levels in a home setting.

CHOOSING THE RIGHT LIVING ARRANGEMENT OPTION

The key decision factors families should use to evaluate living arrangement options are the senior's lifestyle and personal preferences, convenience of the location, appropriateness of the level of care for their stage of decline, and affordability.

Personal preferences often hold more sway than choosing the lowest cost living arrangement option. Some seniors cherish their privacy and larger living quarters, and are happier living alone. Others become lonely living alone in their house, and are happier living and socializing with other seniors in a retirement residence.

Another important factor that often affects the decision is the willingness, capability, and availability of a family member to provide care in their home. As well, a temporary living arrangement option, such as living with a family member or in an assisted-living residence with extra care, may be needed until a nursing-home placement becomes available.

Long-distance caregiving is another reality that may need to be factored in. It can be difficult, frustrating, and stressful to manage care services in a home environment from afar. Without hands-on involvement in person, it is common for medical problems and care-staff performance issues to go undetected. In this case, getting a loved one into a care facility will likely be a better option than hiring care for them in their own home.

Unfortunately, the emotional turmoil that often comes with this life-changing event can cloud judgment. Aging parents may fear change, a loss of independence, and being neglected; adult children may feel guilt, sadness, and hopelessness because they can't protect their parents from elder decline and eventual death.

The decision-making process could also be especially difficult if an emotional tug-of-war erupts between the elder and the primary caregiver, or between the primary caregiver and other family members. A primary caregiver could prefer an option with a more secure environment, for their own peace of mind, or a lighter workload for themselves. An elder, on the other hand, could prefer to live alone or move in with a son or daughter, rather than moving into a nursing home. Openly discussing feelings and concerns is the best way for family members to resolve differences, and make the best decision for all involved.

When clearer heads prevail and careful consideration has been given to the pros and cons of each type of living arrangement, one alternative usually surfaces as the best fit because it:

- provides the appropriate level of care;
- meets lifestyle and personal preferences;
- offers the best option for the elder and primary caregiver;
- can become a comfortable home once the elder's personal belongings have been added; and
- is affordable.

TOP TIPS

Show Respect and Patience

- Uncovering and resolving the fears and concerns of your aging senior, and helping them preserve their dignity and need for self-determination will reduce their resistance to making living arrangement changes.

Know When *No* Means *No*

- If elders are mentally capable, they cannot be placed in a retirement residence or nursing home against their wishes, since they have the legal right to live as they please. Respect their right to make their own decisions.

Help Elder Get into Right Place at Right Time

- If an elder is struggling and their care needs have increased, family members should take on a leadership role, to help them decide which option is best, where their care needs will be met, and their safety will be assured.

- Don't let emotional turmoil that often comes with this type of life-changing event cloud judgment. Openly discussing feelings and concerns is the best way to resolve family differences and make the best decision.

Plan Early for Living Arrangement Changes

- Do research early before a decision has to be made under duress.

- Given the long wait times to get into a nursing home, help elders choose good nursing homes and apply as soon as they reach the dependent-living stage.

Don't Focus on the Name of Seniors' Residences, Focus on the Care

- An independent supportive-living retirement residence does not usually provide all the elements of a supportive-living level of care.
- A memory wing of a retirement residence might sound like the right place for seniors with Alzheimer's disease, but if they have reached the middle stage of the disease and need dependent-living care, a nursing home is a better choice.

Identify Real Cost Differences between Living Arrangement Options

- Include the costs of hiring support services, and the opportunity cost of the use of the family house, when comparing the cost of living at home to a retirement residence.
- Include the costs of a home-care team, respite, and your personal time when comparing the cost of caring for a parent or spouse in your home to an assisted-living residence or nursing home.

9

Finding the Best Retirement Residence with Mom

When I was a young girl, my mother would play a trick called Operation Snappy to get me to help to clean the house before company arrived. She would ask me to choose which chores I wanted to do, rather than whether or not I would help her. Years later, I played the same trick on her, asking her to visit retirement residences with me to get her actively involved in deciding which one she liked best. I hoped that she would change her mind about staying in her house and move to a retirement residence.

Before we started our search, I checked the Yellow Pages for names of retirement residences in Cobourg. As I learned, looking at directories of seniors' care residences would have been more helpful because they are organized by level of care, and usually provide a list of amenities and care services, as well as a picture of the residence and contact information. These directories are available as a stand-alone guide, in seniors' magazines and on-line.

The Care Guide, for example, is available free of charge in Ontario, B.C., and Alberta, at pharmacies, doctor's offices, in hospitals, and other places where seniors typically spend time. The website (www.thecareguide.com) includes listings for Nova Scotia as well. Local branches of the provincial community care agency are another good source of information about seniors' care residences.

Mom and I toured an elegant retirement residence that had once been Victoria College, a degree-granting university in the 1800s. The grand old building, with large private suites and wide bookcase-lined hallways, sits on top of a hill and has a sweeping view of Lake Ontario. Mom was overwhelmed by the immense size of the residence.

Next, we visited a smaller, cozier, and more modern residence, where she could walk to the main street of Cobourg in a few minutes, even with her walker. The resident service manager was informative, helpful, and friendly. We met a charming lady in the lobby who enthusiastically told us that she had just finished sewing some aprons, placemats, and doll clothes for her church bazaar, and couldn't wait to see how well they sold. We asked her how she liked living there. She said she was enjoying her apartment, she felt at home with the staff and other residents, and really had no complaints. Mom, who had been a talented seamstress herself, felt comfortable with her new acquaintance and this particular residence.

In January 2003, my mother took advantage of a one-month trial in a furnished apartment in her preferred retirement residence. Most residences are happy to offer this option. It helps seniors determine if they like the staff, other residents, and the food, and get first-hand experience with the care, laundry, and housekeeping services before moving in all their belongings.

By February, Mom was relieved to be returning home to her beloved red-brick bungalow, where she and Dad had lived for 27 years. A month later, however, she was finding living on her own very difficult and lonely, and she wanted to return to the new friends she had met in the retirement residence. With great relief, Mitch and I quickly found a real estate agent to sell her house.

Moving can be emotionally draining for seniors who are downsizing from a house to a retirement residence and have to part with a lifetime of possessions. It is important that they retain favourite pieces of furniture if they aren't too large, as well as cherished keepsakes and heirlooms, so they won't later regret a hasty decision to sell or give them away. Mom insisted that whatever she couldn't take with her to the retirement residence be given to David or me, or to a friend, neighbour, or a charity.

Used furniture and antique stores, and public auctions can lower stress levels when the contents of a house have to be moved out before new owners move in. The process usually includes appraising, picking up, and then selling household possessions, such as furniture, dishes, collectables, jewellery, pictures, electronics, appliances, and other household articles. Be careful when dealing with auctioneers. David had to make many phone calls to the small-town auctioneer we used before finally receiving the proceeds from the sale. There is also a charge for picking up furniture, and in the larger cities, auctioneers usually only sell high-end furniture.

Less marketable belongings can be given to charities such as the Salvation Army. The Furniture Bank (www.furniturebank. org), is a Toronto-based charity that provides income tax receipts for the value of furniture donated, but it charges for pickups. The Canadian Diabetes Association (www.diabetes.ca) picks up used clothing and household goods, such as dishes, cookware, and towels from front doorsteps of houses, usually free of charge.

For seniors who do not have family, or none that live close enough to help, customized moving services are cropping up to assist them with the downsizing and moving process. Trusted Transitions is a company with several branches in Ontario that can handle all the steps of a move, from planning, sourcing and coordinating movers, to sorting, packing, and unpacking belongings, and then arranging for the sale, donation, disposition, moving, or storing of unwanted household items.

Choosing a retirement residence can be difficult because there is a broad range of amenities, recreational and social activities, and care services offered, and no common way of describing the differences. Apartment formats vary greatly too, from shared accommodations and bachelor or studio suites, to one- and two-bedroom suites with kitchen facilities or kitchenettes.

The level, qualifications, and availability of nursing staff also vary greatly between retirement residences. While many of them have registered or licensed practical nurses on staff, some have a registered nurse, the most skilled nursing level. Other residences don't have any nursing staff. The qualifications of personnel who provide 24-hour emergency response also vary greatly: some retirement residences have registered practical nurses, some have personal support workers, and others have only a responsible person on the night shift. Furthermore, some residences have a visiting doctor, while others do not.

It is therefore very important for families to do their homework when comparing retirement residences. Don't rely only on marketing brochures and magazines, and beware of the seduction of overzealous sales people who promise to be an alternative to a nursing home.

Unlike nursing homes, which are provincially licensed, regulated, and inspected, not all provinces and territories regulate care delivered in retirement residences. In the last five years, B.C., Alberta, Ontario, and Quebec have introduced legislation to govern care in these facilities. The Ontario legislation should be fully in effect by 2012.

Each of these four provinces also has non-profit professional associations for retirement homes. They are the BC Seniors Living Association (BCSLA), the Alberta Senior Citizens' Housing Association (ASCHA), the Ontario Retirement Communities Association (ORCA), and the Regroupement québécois des résidences pour aînés (RQRA) in Quebec. BCSLA and ORCA have developed systems that set standards, inspect, and accredit retirement homes. Many of the directories of seniors' care residences in B.C. and Ontario clearly indicate which retirement residences are approved by these accreditation organizations.

Residents are also covered by whatever landlord-tenant legislation exists in a particular province. If rents are controlled by legislation, then the accommodation portion of monthly fees is controlled. The care services and meals portion of monthly fees, however, are not controlled by this legislation, so residents may experience more price increases in this part of their monthly fees.

Since there is a wide range in the monthly accommodation fees charged, getting fees quoted in writing will help with cost comparisons between retirement residences. Written quotes should clarify what is included in the accommodation fee, what services are available for an additional cost, and what services are not available at all.

Cable television services may or may not be included in monthly fees. Surface or covered parking may be available, and there may or may not be an extra charge. Central air conditioning may be a feature of the residence, but if it is not, there may be a charge to install a window air conditioner in the summer and to remove it in the fall. Also, some retirement residences allow pets, while others don't. If pets are allowed, some retirement residences charge extra each month, while others don't.

A separate schedule should itemize the care services provided for a monthly fee, and the cost of meals. Compare these lists to identify any gaps in care. Retirement homes should also provide a list of additional care services they offer, if any, along with the hourly rates charged for each one. That way, seniors will know what care services are available, and what they will cost, as their health deteriorates.

It is often said that the devil is in the details, so families should carefully read the residency agreement they receive from their chosen retirement residence before signing it. It is important to ensure that this legal contract stipulates that no more than 30 days' written notice is required to terminate the agreement, and that rent increases will be in accordance with the provisions of the Tenant Protection Act, or any successor legislation. The contract should also clarify what residents' options and obligations are, if their health declines and they require nursing care that goes beyond the facility's capability. The agreement should specify whether they can stay, but purchase assisted-living care services, whether they have the right to make arrangements for an external nursing care provider, or whether they must leave. The contract should also stipulate what the options and obligations of both parties are, if a nursing-home placement is not available when needed.

There are four key ingredients that will help families choose a good retirement residence: it's a good fit for the senior; the availability of supportive- and assisted-living care services; professional management and nursing staff; and the building is clean, well-maintained, and safe. See pages 182 to 184 for a list of what to look for and questions to ask when visiting retirement residences.

A GOOD FIT FOR THE SENIOR

It is important that seniors find a retirement residence that is a good fit for them, because this is such a big change from living in their own home. The location of the residence, the compatibility with other residents, and the appearance of the building and the senior's apartment should all make them feel comfortable. Otherwise, they won't be happy living there.

As well, some seniors are unwilling or unable to cook for themselves and like the sociability of dining with other residents. Other seniors, however, prefer and are able to prepare some or all of their meals, so they will live in a residence where they can have a kitchenette in their apartment. These residents may also have higher needs for privacy than more outgoing seniors.

AVAILABILITY OF SUPPORTIVE- AND ASSISTED-LIVING CARE SERVICES

The availability of supportive- and assisted-living care services ensures that seniors will have their increasing care needs met without relocating, unless they reach the dependent-living stage and need to move into a nursing home. Supportive-care services should provide meals, including foods for special diets, snacks, and tray service to apartments if a resident is sick. Weekly housekeeping and laundry, and 24-hour emergency response should also be available. Medications should be administered by a registered or licensed practical nurse, if needed.

Ideally, assisted-living care should include the expertise of a registered nurse to supervise the hands-on nursing care provided by licensed practical nurses. Personal support workers should also be available to help with bathing, dressing, and getting to the dining room, if needed. With an RN, RPNs, and PSWs on staff, a good retirement residence has the professional nursing team in place to handle increasing medical and personal care needs.

PROFESSIONAL MANAGEMENT AND NURSING STAFF

Look for a stable management team that has been in their current positions for several years or more, and registered or licensed practical nurses, certified personal support workers or health-care aides, and an accredited retirement residence in provinces where an accreditation association exists. Ask residents you meet in the hallways if the management team and nursing staff are responsive to their concerns, and whether they are kind and caring. This will be a good indication of the quality of the people.

A CLEAN, WELL-MAINTAINED, AND SAFE BUILDING

Touring not just the lobby and hallways but washrooms, the dining room, and the kitchen will give you a good indication of whether the building is clean and well maintained. If possible, visit a resident's apartment. I visited a friend of our family in his retirement residence, which looked modern, attractive, and in tip-top shape from the appearance of the lobby, dining room, and hallways; however, his kitchenette was so filthy that I felt compelled to disinfect the sink and counters. He certainly wasn't getting his money's worth from what he paid for housekeeping.

Retirement residences should all have an emergency call-bell system in place in residents' rooms and bathrooms, and the building should be monitored 24 hours a day. A fire safety and security system should also be in place that includes a sprinkler system, smoke and heat detectors in residents' rooms and common areas, and security alarms on all exterior doors. There should also be an emergency generator that provides lighting in the event of a power failure.

Elder-proof design features should be in all retirement residences. Look for wheelchair and walker accessible elevators, apartments, and washrooms. Apartments should have grab bars in bathtubs and levered door handles. The building should be well lit throughout, and light switches in apartments should be reachable from wheelchairs.

My mother appeared to be adjusting well to retirement residence life and always seemed to be in a good mood when she was with her friend, Betty. However, several years later I found a prayer that she had written, which broke my heart:

> *Dear Lord,*
>
> *I need you to help me. I feel so sad. I miss Ed and I miss my house and I find it so hard to adjust to everything that has happened to me. My children cannot visit me as often as I would like and I often feel lonely. Thank you for my friend Betty. Please help me to hear better with my new hearing aids and to make new friends, and let me feel your presence with me every day.*
>
> *In Jesus' name. Amen.*

I realized that the grieving process takes longer than I thought. My mother was grieving the loss of her husband and her house, and she was adjusting to a new way of life. What she needed from me was a supportive ear to help her make the transition.

TOP TIPS

Seniors Can Try Out Retirement Residences

- Seniors can take advantage of a one-month trial in a furnished apartment in most retirement residences.

Used Furniture Stores, Public Auctions, and Charities Can Reduce Moving Stress

- When downsizing, used furniture stores and public auctions can sell marketable household items, and charities will take many unmarketable and unwanted belongings.

Know What Is Included in Retirement Residence Fees

- Get written quotes of monthly accommodation fees, listing what is included, what can be added for an additional fee, and what is or isn't allowed, such as pets.
- Get an itemized schedule of care services, listing what is included for the standard monthly fee, and hourly rates charged for additional care services that are offered.
- Compare price lists and level, qualifications, and availability of nursing staff, and identify any gaps in care services between retirement residences.

Understand Options and Obligations of Residency Agreement before Signing

- Ensure contract stipulates that no more than 30 days' written notice is required to terminate the agreement.
- If the senior's health declines beyond the scope of the retirement residence, the agreement must stipulate whether the resident can stay but purchase assisted-living care services, can make arrangements for an external nursing-care provider, or must leave.

What to Look For and Questions to Ask When Visiting Retirement Residences

A Good Fit for the Senior

- Good location, close to friends, family, and community services, such as banks, churches, medical professionals and hospital, good walking routes to shopping, and accessible to public transportation.
- Residents can pick the eating arrangements they prefer—all meals in the dining room or some or all meals prepared in their own private kitchenette.
- Senior feels he or she would be comfortable with other residents.
- Apartment appearance, layout, size, and features, building appearance and ambiance, and social and recreational activities appeal to resident.
- A van takes residents to medical appointments and on outings with other residents.

Availability of Supportive- and Assisted-Living Care Services

Supportive-Living Services

- Meals are provided if desired, including foods for special diets and snacks in dining room, and tray service to apartment if sick.
- Weekly housekeeping of apartments and laundry is provided.
- Emergency response is available 24-hours a day, ideally by a licensed practical nurse.
- Medications are administered by a registered or licensed practical nurse, if needed.

Assisted-Living Care Services

- Ideally, a registered nurse supervises the registered or licensed practical nurses.
- Personal support workers help with personal care, such as bathing, dressing, and getting to the dining room.
- Therapeutic tub is available for residents' use.
- Assisted-living care services are available if needed on an à-la-cart fee basis, or in a separate wing and provided by a care team of a registered nurse, registered practical nurses, and personal support workers.

Professional Management and Nursing Staff

Accredited Retirement Residence

- Look for accredited retirement residences in Quebec, Ontario, Alberta, and B.C.

Stability of Management

- Members of management team have been in their positions for several years.

Professional Nursing Staff

- Registered nurses and registered or licensed practical nurses are all licensed practitioners.
- Personal support workers or health-care aides are certified practitioners.

Positive Feedback from Residents

- Residents say the management and nursing staff are responsive to their concerns.
- There are no morale problems, and staff is kind and caring.

(Continued)

- Residents are pleased with the food and recreational activities.

Clean, Well-Maintained, and Safe Building

Clean and Well-Maintained Building

- Apartments, the kitchen, dining room, activity rooms, washrooms, stairwells, and exterior grounds look clean and well maintained.
- Heating, ventilation, and air conditioning are available in apartments and common areas, and individually controlled in apartments.

Safety Measures in Place

- An emergency call-bell system exists in residents' bedrooms and bathrooms, and is centrally monitored 24 hours a day.
- Building fire safety system meets government fire codes, has a sprinkler system, and is monitored 24 hours a day.
- Smoke and heat detectors are in residents' rooms and common areas.
- Security alarms exist on all exterior doors of the building.
- Emergency generator provides lighting in the event of a power failure.

Elder-Proof Design Features

- Elevators, apartments, and all washrooms are wheelchair and walker accessible.
- Residence has low-pile carpets, wide corridors, and levered door handles.
- Apartment washrooms have high toilet seats and grab bars.
- The building is well lit throughout and light switches in apartments are reachable from wheelchairs.

(10)

Finding a Good Nursing Home for Mom

For 14 years, when Doris was in her 60s and 70s, she volunteered with the pastoral care program of St. Peter's Anglican Church. She visited elders in one of the Cobourg nursing homes and grew especially attached to a very independent-minded woman named Mrs. Hartwick, who at first didn't want any company. She soon grew to enjoy visits from her new friend. When Mrs. Hartwick died at the grand old age of 102, Doris was sad for days. The residents so loved Doris' fun-loving demeanour, and her friendly Newfoundland accent, that the nursing-home staff often requested her help with special events and she was always very obliging.

Back then, Mom said on several occasions, "I don't ever want to end up living in a nursing home myself." She feared them because she thought they were a place where people go to die. I think she irrationally surmised that as long as she could avoid living in one she wouldn't die.

It was with this vivid tormented flashback, in February 2004, that I absorbed the news from a hospital discharge planner that my mother needed to apply for a nursing-home placement. The retirement residence where Mom had lived for only five months couldn't take her back, because her nursing care needs went beyond the level of care available there.

I learned that elders must apply to their local community care agency for a nursing-home placement. Each province has its own name for these agencies but you can find them by calling the Regional Health Authority responsible for your community. In Ontario, they are called Local Health Integration Networks and the community care agency in charge of nursing homes is called the Community Care Access Centre (CCAC).

Once seniors apply, they will be assessed, and if they qualify, placed on waiting lists for their preferred nursing homes. A case manager with CCAC in Cobourg came to the hospital and assessed my mother's physical and mental capabilities. Her nursing-home application also included an assessment by a medical doctor. I was told very definitively that she had reached the dependent-living stage and qualified to live in a nursing home.

If Doris had been declared mentally capable of making her own decisions, she would have had to sign her consent on her nursing-home application form. In that case, the hospital discharge planner, David, and I would have discussed with Mom living arrangement options available to her, so that she could have made an informed decision. However, because she was deemed mentally incompetent, I signed her application form, giving consent as her substitute decision-maker. I did this only after making the difficult decision with David to place her in an "old folks" home.

The discharge planner, who acted as an agent for CCAC, requested that I quickly choose a maximum of three nursing homes so that Mom could be placed on a waiting list for each one as soon as possible; the maximum in Ontario has since changed to five and maximums may vary by province. Wait times could be as long as three or four years for the highest demand nursing homes and if applying for basic accommodations. If a senior applies for the maximum allowable nursing homes, some lower-demand nursing homes, or can afford a semi-private or private room, the wait time could be considerably less. Wait times will vary greatly by area and province.

According to the Ontario Long-Term Care Homes Act, the highest priority placements in nursing homes go to elders who clinically qualify to be in a nursing home, and are in a crisis situation. This emergency may arise from their condition or circumstances, such as living alone, and having no spouse, family, or friends to support them. The next highest priority placements are elders who qualify to be in a nursing home, are in a hospital but no longer need hospital care, and the hospital is experiencing severe capacity pressure, or is closing some or all of their beds.

The wait times for ailing elders who live at home with other family members, and those in retirement residences or hospitals without capacity problems or closures could therefore be much longer, unless they become very ill and in need of an immediate placement. In that case, they would be bumped up to a level one priority. Each province has regulations that govern nursing homes, so the priority of placements may vary somewhat.

With overwhelming feelings of guilt and betrayal, David and I made it our personal mission to find the very best nursing home for Mom. I received the names of the nursing homes in the area from the CCAC, then I asked my mother's friends, neighbours, and the parish nurse from her church to divulge any local knowledge about these nursing homes, good or bad.

I found five prospective nursing homes with an Alzheimer's Unit and we called the administrator of each one to learn more and arrange a tour. I learned afterwards that David, Mitch, and I should have visited the ones we liked best several times to see if our impression of the facility and staff remained the same. We should have met the administrator and had a tour on a weekday, and returned unannounced, at a different time of day on a weekend, when there may have been fewer nursing employees on duty.

As we entered the first facility, I felt very sad because my mother needed this high level of care and wouldn't get any better. I feared that she would be neglected amongst a sea of sick people. I also felt tremendously guilty that I hadn't decided to bring an army of nurses, 24 hours a day, into my home to care for her instead. However, I realized this option would be cost prohibitive, and would make it impossible for me to keep working. It would also have been a very isolated life for Mom, compared to living in a nursing home surrounded by many people.

Once I started to look at elders who appeared to have dementia, I instinctively thought my mother did not belong in a nursing home, because her cognitive impairment didn't seem as severe to me. The sight of an impatient-looking man loudly banging his spoon on a dining room table disturbed me. I also saw a rosy-cheeked, dark-haired woman, likely only in her 60s, lying lifelessly in a tilt-back wheelchair. A personal support worker was busy trying to feed her pureed food that looked like coloured mush. Mom still had much more life in her.

It took me about a month after Mom moved into her nursing home to realize that I had been in denial about her disabilities. I needed an adjustment period to get to know other residents and I soon learned to look beyond the ruthless disintegration of human bodies and minds. I discovered that the man who made the ruckus with his spoon was just looking for attention. When a personal support worker passed him a newspaper he became so absorbed in it that he took on the persona of a young businessman. To my delight, I discovered the special person that each elder had been and still was, and I comprehended that my mother was indeed in the right place.

We discovered that two of the five long-term care homes were not at all as depressing as the media and our mother would have us believe. They appeared to be very professionally operated, the staff showed concern, respect, and compassion for residents, and treated them as individuals. The buildings were modern, attractive, clean, and inviting. These care homes were places that David, Mitch, and I felt would provide a comfortable and safe home for Mom and a pleasant environment for all of us. These nursing homes did not resemble the sterile institutions and acute-care hospitals of 20 years ago. Since then, the push has been on to create a comfortable home environment, acknowledging that these buildings become the home of the residents who live there. In Ontario, the name of nursing homes has officially been changed from *long-term care facilities* to *long-term care homes*, reflecting this new direction.

There were a few nursing homes, however, that did depress and even shock us. In one facility we found dingy and poorly lit hallways, low ceilings, and washroom entrances in hallways rather than in residents' rooms. In another facility, the smell of urine permeated the hallways in the residents' quarters. The dining room was on a different floor, so there were long line-ups of residents waiting for personal support workers to take them on the one elevator to the dining room. It looked as if residents were being warehoused in this particular building. I vowed that my mother would never set foot in any of these establishments.

We chose two nursing homes that we agreed would be good enough for Mom. We didn't put a third choice on her application form, because we couldn't find another nursing home in the area with which we felt comfortable.

The key ingredients of good nursing homes are professional and caring management and nursing staff, and strong family support. When these are in place, there are three positive outcomes for residents: good health and hygiene care; an enhanced quality of life; and a clean, safe, and well-maintained building.

A Good Nursing Home

Key Ingredients

Professional and Caring Management & Nursing Staff	Strong Family Support

Key Outcomes

Good Health & Hygiene Care

Enhanced Quality of Life

Clean, Safe, & Well-Maintained Building

KEY INGREDIENTS OF A GOOD NURSING HOME

Professional and Caring Management and Nursing Staff

The quality of the management and the nursing staff is more important in nursing homes than retirement residences, because frail residents, who have serious illnesses, are so much more vulnerable and dependent on them for their well-being. Therefore, professional and caring management and nursing staff is the crucial ingredient that separates good nursing homes from middle-of-the road and below-average nursing facilities.

In good nursing homes, management and nursing staff are disciplined, well organized, and very skilled. They also care passionately about elderly people, and are responsive and attentive to their individual needs. Their job means so much more to them than just picking up a paycheque. It is obvious to family members and visitors that these managers and nursing employees are glad to work there and they work well as a team. Their respect and kindness for residents is evident because they call each one by their name, and when called, happy recognition of the staff member shows on the residents' faces.

The administrator and director of nursing, also called director of care, have the most influence on the performance of the nursing home, and ultimately on the care and well-being of residents. Frequent turnover in these positions can lead to inconsistent leadership, low staff morale, and below-average resident care. Ideally, they should have been in their current position for two or more years.

These are the key people that families should meet to see if they are approachable, and make them comfortable with their management style. Ask residents and their families, who you meet in the hallways, whether the administrator and director of nursing are involved in their care and are responsive to their concerns. Learn as much as possible about these managers, including their background experience. If you get a bad feeling about them, then it may be best to eliminate that nursing home from your list.

Long-term care homes are licensed and regulated by provincial government laws, service contracts, and by standards and policies. Their current provincial government licence should be posted somewhere in their front entrance reception area or hallway. Nursing homes are inspected annually, and more often, if there are complaints of non-compliance. When this happens, nursing homes are given a specified period of time to address the problem or problems. A nursing home's licence can be suspended for continued non-compliance. Families should ask the administrator for the most recent provincial government inspection findings, and the actions that have been taken to correct any deficiencies. This will be a telling indication of a nursing home's performance, and the administrator's willingness to communicate with families.

The Long-Term Care Homes Act in each province dictates that nursing homes develop a care plan for each resident that articulates proposed goals, planned care, and clear directions to nursing staff and others who will be providing care. On one occasion, I reviewed and requested minor changes to my mother's care plan. I was impressed that she was essentially getting care tailored for her illnesses, risks, personality, and likes and dislikes.

The new Ontario legislation that came into effect July 1, 2010, stipulates that the preparation of the care plan requires the involvement of the resident, their substitute decision-maker for personal care, if there is one, and any other person that the resident or substitute decision-maker wishes to assist them. These plans must be assessed for effectiveness and revised, if required, at least every six months.

In the better nursing homes, the director of nursing hires more full-time than part-time staff, and does not hire contract workers. That way, the same shift team of registered practical nurses and personal support workers care for the same residents for four to five days a week.

The management in good nursing homes encourages family involvement. The director of care invites residents and their family to an annual care conference with all their department heads. Mom and I never missed one, and David called in on speakerphone from Vancouver. This is a good opportunity to build an alliance with the key people who take care of your loved one, to hear their perspectives on your parent or spouse's health status, and to collectively find solutions to any unresolved issues.

Good nursing-home management teams also encourage and support the establishment of family or resident councils, whose main purpose is to protect and improve the quality of life of residents. Additionally, these councils give families and residents a voice in decisions that affect them.

Strong Family Support

Residents receive better care when families and friends visit often and are involved in their care and well-being. When families fail to take an interest in the care of their loved one, it is only human nature that nursing staff may become complacent, and provide only the minimum care necessary. If families don't care, why should they? However, good nursing homes can become great nursing homes when families:

- notice and show their appreciation to nursing staff that go the extra mile in caring for their loved ones;
- become involved in their loved ones' care and help to meet their comfort, social, emotional, intellectual, and spiritual needs; and
- notice and express concern to the nursing management or administrator if they witness neglect or poor nursing care of their loved ones.

Residents benefit most when families and nursing-home staff work together to meet their care and quality-of-life needs. This means that the resident and their substitute decision-maker attend annual care conferences, and review and approve medications and the care plan, when it is updated every six months. They also discuss any newly arising health issues with the registered nurse or registered practical nurse. Arranging for volunteer companions or hired caregiver-companions can also greatly improve the life of residents, because family caregivers usually can't visit their loved one every day. If they do, they won't have a life of their own.

I have a friend who worked in management positions in nursing homes for many years. She told me that when residents have family and friends who listen attentively to them and demonstrate their love, they are much happier, socialize more with other residents, feel more secure, have higher self-esteem, and are less often depressed.

When nursing homes work well, they become a tightly knit community of residents, their families, and employees from all departments. My mother and I got to know many of the people who worked in her nursing home—the managers, nursing staff in the Alzheimer's unit, physiotherapists, activities coordinator, laundry manager, dietitian, chef, cleaning staff, and the maintenance man. We needed them all, and they became part of our extended family that helped to keep Mom happy and well cared for.

KEY OUTCOMES FOR RESIDENTS

Good Health and Hygiene Care

Good nursing homes have adequate nursing staff to handle the care needs of their residents. The lower the ratio of nursing staff to residents that you see on a particular floor in a nursing home the more attentive is the care. There should be, on average, one personal support worker for every 10 residents for the day and evening shifts, and one PSW for every 16 residents on the night shift. The ratio in Alzheimer's units during the day and evening shifts ought to be slightly lower, about 1 to 8.

The ratio of registered practical nurses should be, on average, 1 for every 32 residents on a 24-hour-a-day basis. There should also be a full-time registered nurse on duty at all times who can handle the needs of approximately 130 residents. Ideally, a director of care, an assistant director of care, and a wound-care specialist, who are all registered nurses, should also be available for eight hours a day, five days a week.

It is easy to tell if residents are receiving good hygiene care: they look clean, well groomed, and appropriately dressed for the season and time of day. To minimize the risk of spreading viruses and bacterial infections, residents' hands and fingernails should be cleaned often, and their fingernails should be cut short. There should be no persistently strong odours of urine or feces permeating the residents' quarters or the dining rooms.

Residents should be given a bath twice a week, but legislation in some provinces may stipulate a minimum of only once a week. They should be receiving a sponge bath on the other days, and getting their hair and teeth brushed at least daily, and nail care twice a week, if they are unable to complete these personal-care duties on their own.

Nursing-home residents should have access to a primary care physician, who visits the nursing home at least once a week. They should also be on call for them, usually by phone, in case of an emergency, or when they need a new medication. Physiotherapists should be working regularly with residents, if they have restricted movement or are recovering from broken bones. As well, a dentist should be visiting once a month to handle routine dental care.

Enhanced Quality of Life

Appetizing, tasty, and nutritious food is crucial for the health and well-being of residents. Daily menus offering two meal options should be posted in dining rooms. Check to see if they offer variety and balance. Staying for a lunch or dinner makes sense to ensure the food is fresh, and tastes, smells, and looks appetizing. Personal support workers seen helping some residents eat, especially in the Alzheimer's unit, ought to be a common occurrence. As well, a dietitian should be involved in meal planning to address residents' nutritional problems as their health declines.

Families who are in the process of selecting a nursing home ought to glance into residents' rooms to see if they have a cheerful decor and a window. There should be storage space for their personal belongings, and room for their own telephone and TV. The presence of residents in the common areas during the day should be a familiar scene, rather than seeing them alone in their rooms.

Activity calendars ought to be prominently posted on bulletin boards throughout nursing homes. They should include a wide range of activities to stimulate residents' minds, bodies, and souls, including exercise, music, entertainment, seasonal events, and religious services. Seeking out the activities coordinator is a good idea to find out if they take residents to activities and spend one-on-one personal time with each of them.

Inviting common areas ought to exist for dining, socializing, activities, and special entertainment events. Ideally, there will also be private comfortable areas for families to spend time or share a meal with their loved ones.

Clean, Safe, and Well-Maintained Building

Cleanliness is of utmost importance in nursing homes because infections can easily spread among residents. Residents' rooms, floors, dining rooms, hallways, handrails, washrooms, and kitchens should be cleaned every day. I was thankful that the administrator was a real stickler for cleanliness, and it showed. If you don't see cleaning staff working while on your tour you should ask how often the residents' quarters are cleaned. It is also important to see if the residents' rooms, washrooms, and common areas look to be in good repair.

Heating, ventilation, and air conditioning should all be controlled on each floor and in the residents' rooms, because most nursing-home buildings have several floors. Mom lived on the ground floor, so it could be cooler there than on the second floor, and yet, sometimes on very hot summer days it could be sweltering on her floor, because the air-conditioning system didn't always work well.

Building safety is crucial in nursing homes, because there are so many frail and disabled people to evacuate in an emergency.

Smoking should not be permitted anywhere in the building. These facilities should have smoke detectors, sprinklers, and an alarm system, and management should regularly conduct fire drills and have an evacuation plan. Touring families ought to ask the administrator if there is a backup generator to provide lighting in the event of a power failure. A secured front entrance and medical response call bells, located beside residents' beds and in all washrooms, are mandatory in nursing homes.

See pages 200 to 204 for a list of what to look for and questions to ask when visiting nursing homes.

In early April 2004, David received a call from the CCAC offering Mom a private room in a nursing home that was just opening. Her waiting time was only two months for three reasons. First, she was coming from a hospital that was experiencing severe capacity pressure, so she was rated the second highest priority for a nursing-home placement. Second, she was offered a placement in a new nursing home that was just opening its doors. Third, she was applying for a private room. Wait times are usually much shorter for private and semi-private rooms, compared to basic accommodations.

We were given 24 hours to accept the offer. Although this nursing home was our second-choice, we felt very comfortable with it, and readily accepted the offer. Had we declined, Mom's file would have been closed, and the offer would then have been made to another person on the same day. In that case, Mom would have had to wait six months before reapplying, unless her circumstances or medical condition got much worse, indicating that she was in a crisis situation.

Ontario regulations limit bed-holding to five days. Once we accepted the offer, we had two days to move our mother in, or pay a bed-holding fee for an additional three days. If we both had been away, and couldn't move our mother in within six days from the day we received the offer, then we would have lost the placement. Other provinces may have different timelines and penalties.

David flew in from Vancouver straight away to move our mother into her new home. I happened to be on vacation at the time, but I returned to Toronto a few days later and rushed to the nursing home where I was able to help one of the registered nurses complete Mom's care plan, by providing information about her medical history. The plan should have been completed within 24 hours of admittance, but because there were so many residents moving in at the same time it hadn't been finished yet.

About nine months later, the CCAC offered Doris a room in the nursing home that had been our first choice, but we turned it down because we were happy with our choice. Doris' nursing-home care team was very responsive to any concerns that we raised, and they understood and treated her very well. Importantly, it would have been very upsetting for Mom to go through the stress of another move.

Families should expect an adjustment period when their loved one first moves into a nursing home. Fear, anxiety, and depression are common until residents get settled into their new home. Doris was frightened at first, but with time she grew very comfortable with her room, with the nursing staff, her caregiver-companions, and with the other residents. In a care conference a year later, the director of nursing asked Mom if she liked living there. She smiled warmly and said yes, without any hesitation.

After spending time in a good nursing home for five years with Mom, I learned that while they are a good place to die, they are an even better place to live. Evidence of life is everywhere. Residents can be seen talking, watching TV and listening to music, smiling, laughing, singing, clapping their hands, exercising, eating and helping to clear the dining room tables, walking through hallways and gardens, and yes, napping in the middle of the afternoon. I am no longer apprehensive about nursing homes. I realize that a good nursing home is often the right living arrangement at the dependent-living and palliative-care stages of decline.

TOP TIPS

Scout Early for the Best Nursing Homes

- Investigate nursing-home options early, while an elder is still well, but starting to decline. That way, if they have a medical emergency and urgently need a placement, no time will be lost deciding which nursing homes are the best to put on the application form.

Uncover Local Knowledge about Nursing Home Performance

- Ask administrator for the results of their nursing home's most recent government inspection reports and verified complaints, and what actions have been taken to correct deficiencies.
- Tap into the local intelligence of friends, neighbours, charities, churches, doctors, and nurses to find out which nursing homes families and their loved ones like, and dislike.

Accepting a Private or Semi-Private Room Can Shorten Wait Times

- Semi-private and private rooms cost approximately $250 to $550 more a month than basic accommodations, but can substantially shorten an elder's wait time for a nursing home, and give them more space and privacy.

Good People are the Key Ingredient of the Best Nursing Homes

- Professional and caring management and nursing staff ensure that residents obtain good health and hygiene care and an enhanced quality of life, and live in a clean, safe, and well-maintained building.

The Administrator and Director of Nursing Are the Leaders of Nursing Homes

- The administrator and director of nursing have the most influence over the care and well-being of residents, and should be involved in their care. If you don't have confidence in these key people, choose another nursing home.

Strong Family Support Can Turn Good Nursing Homes into Great Nursing Homes

- Residents receive better care when their family visits often and is involved in their care and well-being.

Nursing-Home Communications Tools Ensure Well-Coordinated Care

- Care plans articulate goals, planned care, and clear directions to nursing staff for each resident. They must be updated at least every six months, and involve the input of residents and their substitute decision-maker.

- A care conference builds an alliance between family and health-care professionals, and can help find solutions to unresolved problems.

What to Look For and Questions to Ask When Touring Nursing Homes

Professional and Caring Management and Nursing Staff

Accreditation

- Nursing home posts a current licence from a provincial government.

Correction of Deficiencies

- Administrator makes available copy of the most recent deficiency list, and outlines actions already taken to correct deficiencies, if there are any.

High Calibre and Stable Management

- Administrator and director of nursing are involved in the care of each resident, have extensive experience, and have been in their current position for two or more years.

Professional Nursing Staff

- Care plans are developed and updated at least every six months, so each resident receives care tailored for their individual needs.
- Care conferences are conducted annually with residents and their family.

Positive Culture

- Staff appears happy to work there and works well as a team.

Residents Are Treated with Kindness and Respect

- Staff demonstrate kindness and compassion toward residents, and treat them as individuals, and with respect and dignity.
- Employees call residents by name and are recognized by them.
- Family or resident councils are up and running.

Good Health and Hygiene Care

Adequate Level of Nursing Staff

- A full-time registered nurse is on duty at all times.
- The average ratio of personal support workers to residents is 1 to 10 during the day and evening shifts, and 1 to 16 on the night shift.
- In a dementia wing the ratio is 1 to 8 during the day and evening shifts.
- The average ratio of registered practical nurses to residents is 1 to 32 on all shifts.

Residents Receive Good Hygiene Care

- Residents look clean, well groomed, and appropriately dressed for the season and time of day.
- Residents' hair and teeth are brushed at least once a day.
- Residents' hands and fingernails are washed often and their fingernails are cut short.
- There are no persistently strong odours of urine or feces permeating the residents' quarters or the dining room.
- Residents have a bath twice a week and a sponge bath on other days.

(Continued)

Access to Other Health-Care Professionals

- A primary care physician visits at least once a week, and is on call for residents.
- Physiotherapists and a therapy room are available on-site.
- A dentist visits monthly.

Enhanced Quality of Life

Food is Appetizing, Tasty, and Nutritious

- Daily menus are posted in dining room and appear to provide variety and balanced meals.
- Two meal options are available to residents.
- Food tastes, looks, and smells appetizing, is fresh, and at the appropriate temperature.
- Personal support workers are seen helping some residents eat.
- A dietitian addresses nutritional problems as health declines.

Residents' Rooms Have Personal Touches and Provide Privacy

- Personal belongings and a few pieces of furniture are allowed in residents' rooms.
- Rooms have bright cheerful decor and a window.
- Residents can have their own telephone and TV in their room, and there is storage space for their clothes and other belongings.
- Privacy curtains are installed and used, if a bedroom is shared.
- There is a process for switching roommates, if roommates don't get along.

- To preserve their privacy, residents aren't seen being bathed, dressed, or toileted.

Comfortable Amenities

- Cheerful and inviting common areas exist for dining, socializing, activities, and special entertainment events.
- Private comfortable areas exist for families to spend time with their loved ones.

Social and Recreational Activities Are Readily Available

- Monthly activities calendar is sent to residents and their family and prominently posted.
- Events coordinators spend one-on-one time with residents and take them to activities.
- Pleasant outdoor areas with gardens exist.
- Most residents are with other residents in the common areas during the day.

Clean, Safe, and Well-Maintained Home

Clean and Well-Maintained Residents' Rooms and Building

- Residents' rooms, floors, hallways, handrails, dining rooms, washrooms, and kitchen are cleaned daily, and are in good repair.
- Facility should be at a comfortable temperature and have fresh air circulating.

Safety and Security Measures in Place

- Smoking is not permitted anywhere in the building.

(Continued)

- Nursing home has smoke detectors, sprinklers, and an alarm system, regularly conducts fire drills, and has an evacuation plan.
- Emergency generator provides lighting in the event of a power failure.
- Building has a secured front entrance.
- Medical response call bells are located beside residents' beds and in bathrooms.
- Hallways have continuous handrails and are wide enough for two wheelchairs.
- Bathrooms have grab bars.

(11)

Dealing with Dementia

The brain is the command centre for the entire body, and is the most complex and least understood vital organ. As a result, there are many debilitating brain disorders that have no known cause, prevention, or cure.

Dementia is a brain disorder characterized by a progressive deterioration of thinking ability and memory that is severe enough to interfere with daily functioning. According to the Alzheimer Society of Canada, the illness affects approximately half a million Canadians, and the incidence of dementia is expected to escalate as baby boomers reach their senior years, and as medical advances in other areas extend their lives.

Alzheimer's disease is the most common cause of dementia, accounting for approximately 60 per cent of all cases. Lewy body dementia is another common form of the disease, which can develop in advanced stages of Parkinson's disease. A stroke often damages brain tissue and can lead to another common form of dementia called vascular dementia. Huntington's disease leads to cognitive decline and dementia as well.

Alzheimer's disease damages and eventually destroys brain cells. As each area of the brain is affected, people living with the disease lose more of their mental functions, such as their ability to remember, reason, make decisions, speak, and perform familiar tasks. Over time, the brain shrinks significantly, along with loss of brain functions. Eventually, the disease causes total disability and death. The specific causes of Alzheimer's disease are still under investigation, and there is no known cure.

The highest incidence of Alzheimer's disease is among seniors over the age of 65, with one in three developing the disease after the age of 85. While the incidence is low, people can start to develop the illness in their 40s or 50s.

My mother and aunt have both struggled with Alzheimer's disease and I spent three years on the national board of Parkinson Society Canada. My intimate exposure to these mind-altering and relentlessly debilitating brain disorders has turned me into a fighter.

I did not give into my feelings of grief, bewilderment, and helplessness as I watched my mother slowly slip away from me, all the while knowing that I couldn't stop the ruthless invasion of her brain. Instead, I have searched for a better understanding of degenerative neurological diseases, and for coping mechanisms to make life easier for our family. Writing this book and sharing my learning is part of my arsenal to defeat these wicked chronic illnesses that can have a stranglehold on families for a decade or more.

According to a *Mayo Clinic Health Solutions* article "Alzheimer's Disease, New Research Brings Hope," "while medications can help, caregiving is at the heart of Alzheimer's treatment."[1] The same holds true for other forms of dementia. This chapter provides guidance to families so they can have a better journey with dementia. The three areas of advice are based on information I received from the Alzheimer Society, as well as lessons that I have learned while caring for my mother.

1. Obtain an early diagnosis and develop a plan.

2. Gain an understanding of the disease progression.

3. Learn caregiving strategies for a higher quality of life together.

---

[1] "Alzheimer's Disease, New Research Brings Hope," Supplement to Mayo Clinic Health Letter, *Mayo Clinic Health Solutions*, October 2008.

OBTAIN AN EARLY DIAGNOSIS
AND DEVELOP A PLAN

When my mother started to have memory problems, I thought that short-term lapses in memory were common in older people. I have since learned that cognitive problems severe enough to interfere with daily living are not a normal part of aging. I noticed several of the early warning signs of Alzheimer's disease a few months after my father died, in November 2002. Mom would call me two or three times a day to ask the same question over and over again. At that time, the calls seemed to be an intrusion into my busy life. I thought she just needed time to adjust to living alone.

However, my mother also needed help to remember to take her medications and she was constantly losing things. My very sociable mother seemed to be withdrawing from her friends and neighbours. At first, I mistakenly thought her depression was an outgrowth of grief; however, when a neighbour reported that Mom no longer recognized her I realized something was terribly wrong.

Families who suspect a loved one may be developing Alzheimer's disease or another form of dementia should watch for problems in three areas: memory loss, mood changes, and uncharacteristic behaviour. The following warning signs are a summary of information I received from the Alzheimer Society of Canada, as well as my own observations.

Early Warning Signs of Alzheimer's Disease

Type of Problem	Warning Signs
Memory Loss	• Repeating same story or asking same question over and over again • Forgetting to take medications, keep appointments, or do chores • Forgetting names of familiar people and important information • Forgetting simple words or subtituting words *(Continued)*

Type of Problem	Warning Signs
Mood Changes	• Depression or sadness for no apparent reason • Atypical anger and frustration
Uncharacteristic Behaviour	• Misplacing things and putting them in strange places, such as a frying pan in a freezer • Losing interest in favourite activities and initiative to get things done • Neglecting personal hygiene, grooming, and appearance • Getting lost driving or driving poorly

By February 2003, Mom's symptoms became more disabling so I couldn't deny her problem any longer. By that time, her sister in Ottawa had been diagnosed with mild dementia at the age of 90. She had been placed on a medication to slow the progression of the disease. After six months, her memory had not deteriorated and she had not experienced any side effects.

I discussed the medication and my aunt's stabilization with my mother and she agreed to talk to her doctor about it on her next visit. Since I lived in a different city, I sent her primary care physician a letter expressing my concern that my mother might be in the early stage of dementia. I didn't know anything about Alzheimer's disease back then, but I correctly associated abnormal memory loss with dementia.

In my letter, I asked the doctor if he thought a medication might delay the progression of dementia, and if so, if he could arrange to have her tested, and put on a medication if warranted. I also advised him that my mother would like to discuss this matter with him on her next appointment, which was just a week away. Mom's good friend Sue accompanied her to her doctor's appointment and took notes so I would know the outcome.

Mom's family doctor referred her to a geriatric psychiatrist. He could have made the diagnosis himself if he was comfortable doing so, or referred her to a geriatrician or a neurologist, depending on which specialists were available in the Cobourg area. A referral to a memory disorder clinic would have been another good option for an early diagnosis, medications, and follow-up.

The geriatric psychiatrist conducted a mini-mental state examination (MMSE), which is one of a number of commonly used screening tests for dementia and mental competency. He confirmed dementia and put my mother on a medication. At that time, I did not know that there were different types of dementia.

Looking back, I wish I had known to request my mother's test results, a more specific diagnosis of the type of dementia that she had, what stage of the disease she was in, and what disease progression to expect. I only learned that my mother had Alzheimer's disease years later, when we asked her nursing-home doctor to complete a form to apply for a disability tax credit.

I also regret not openly discussing my concerns with my mother when they first arose, so that she could have obtained an earlier diagnosis and treatment. Seeing a primary care physician as soon as symptoms are detected, and getting a physical exam, diagnosis, and a treatment plan are very important for a number of reasons.

If a person is diagnosed with Alzheimer's disease, medications designed to slow the progression of the disease work best when taken in the early stages of the illness. Developing a treatment plan with a primary care physician helps the person feel more in control of this overpowering disease. Taking action also gives hope for a disease where there is little hope of a cure in their lifetime.

An early diagnosis is also important, so that the person and their family will be able to plan for the time when he or she is no longer able to make his or her own decisions, take care of himself or herself, and eventually need round-the-clock care. Having a will in place, and appointing substitute decision-makers for personal care and property should be taken care of right away. These legal documents can't be completed once a parent or spouse is deemed mentally incompetent.

Knowing early on will also give the person and their family the chance to plan for life with dementia, and address the challenges they will face together. It is the best time, while dementia is not too advanced, to discuss care options and the wishes of the person with the disease. Discussions should include what quality of life means to them in terms of their values and preferences. Their views on using feeding tubes should also be made known, because in the late stage of dementia this may be a decision that families have to make on their behalf. These discussions will guide family caregivers in the years ahead.

This is also a good time to talk about difficult issues, such as the eventual necessity to stop driving, and under what circumstances it will be the right time to move into a care facility. This will reduce the torment on caregivers later on when they must do what is in their loved one's best interest, rather than give in to their demands for continued independence.

The Alzheimer Society has First Link® coordinators who families can call at the beginning of their dementia journey when they most need advice and help to cope with the diagnosis. Each chapter of the organization across Canada offers educational programs and information about the disease, teaches coping skills and care strategies, and runs support groups for people with dementia and for their family caregivers.

The health charity's website (www.alzheimer.ca) is also a great place to start to learn the basics about Alzheimer's disease. Another good website is http://onmemory.ca, which was developed in consultation with the Alzheimer Society of Canada and is dedicated to helping caregivers get started.

GAIN AN UNDERSTANDING OF THE DISEASE PROGRESSION

It is important for the person with dementia and their family to gain an understanding of the progression of the particular type of dementia that they have. This will help them plan for the type of help they will eventually need, and prepare emotionally for what lies ahead. Each type of dementia has its own unique progression, sequence of declining abilities, and average duration. I'm using

Alzheimer's disease in my example of disease progression because it is the most common form of the disorder, and affects all areas of the brain.

Alzheimer's disease can last for 3 to 20 years, but on average lasts for 8 to 12 years. My mother had the disease for seven years, but she didn't exhibit symptoms until later in life, at the age of 84. This unrelenting illness has three distinguishable stages of decline: early, middle, and late. In each stage, the four areas of decline that may occur are: cognitive deficits, mood and emotional changes, uncharacteristic behaviour, and physical problems.

The disease progression, in terms of the decline in abilities and length of time at each stage is unique to each person. Which symptoms will actually appear and the order in which they appear will also vary from person to person. Symptoms will also fluctuate for each person. There will be good and bad days and better times of day, most often when a person is more rested.

People living with Alzheimer's disease are, however, able to remember things and people from long ago much longer than they can remember recent events and people in their lives today. Unless there is early damage to the frontal lobe area of the brain, social graces tend to last longer than judgment.

Early Stage: Period of Disease Awareness and Frustration

I call the early stage the period of awareness and frustration as people living with Alzheimer's disease recognize their growing limitations. This is also the stage when family caregivers usually are the most impatient with their loved one, because they aren't yet accustomed to dealing with someone who has dementia.

The symptoms described in the three tables that follow are for each stage of the disease. The summaries were developed from information I received from the Alzheimer Society of Canada, including "By Us for Us" guides written by people

Early Stage: Period of Disease Awareness and Frustration

Areas of Decline	Symptoms that May Occur
Cognitive Deficits	**Memory** • Short-term memory decline, such as forgetting names, location of objects, and taking their medications • Forgetting to turn off the stove and lights • Difficulty learning anything new • Forgetting what was just read or not reading every word **Communications** • Difficulty finding right words or at a loss for words • Losing train of thought easily • Have difficulty following or keeping up with a conversation, especially when people speak quickly **Reasoning** • Aware of declining ability • Thinking tasks take longer than they did before • Difficulty handling money matters and following directions • Confused about dates • Impaired ability to reason and make sound decisions
Mood & Emotions	• Mood swings • Depressed or sad • Frustrated by declining abilities
Uncharacteristic Behaviour	• Passiveness and withdrawal from usual activities and people • Difficulty concentrating, short attention span • Restlessness and wandering • Agitated, confused, suspicious, or indifferent
Physical Problems	• Mild coordination problems • Declining proficiency handling personal care • Declining driving proficiency

with early-stage dementia, from the book *Gentlecare* by Moyra Jones, and from my personal observations of people living with the disease.

Wandering is a common behaviour for people living with Alzheimer's disease that may start in the early stage of the disease, and usually occurs when a person is trying to find a familiar place that feels safer than their current surroundings; however, they may get lost when the way home becomes temporarily unfamiliar to them. Combined with an impaired ability to reason and make sound judgments, this behaviour can lead to injury or even death from exposure or drowning.

Loved ones who have the potential to become lost while walking or driving should be registered with the Alzheimer Society's Safely Home® program. The society collects vital information about registrants, which is held in the RCMP's computer database and is accessible by police forces across North America. For a small fee, the health charity gives registered people a bracelet to wear on their wrist, which has their identification number and instructions to call the police if they are found. If a loved one has lost their way, their family notifies the local police detachment so they can try to find them and return them safely home.

Usually in the early stage, another critical fork in the road is determining when it is no longer safe to drive. According to the Alzheimer Society, "Alzheimer's disease and other related dementias cause changes that affect a person's ability to drive a motor vehicle safely. However, people with this disease may be capable of driving safely for some time after the diagnosis, depending on the timing of the diagnosis and the rate at which the disease progresses."

The society recommends ongoing monitoring of the person's driving ability by family members. When unsafe driving has been witnessed they should discuss the matter with the person and their doctor. Physicians are required by law in some provinces, and by professional ethics, to report to provincial licensing authorities any medical conditions that could impair a person's ability to drive.

Middle Stage: Emotional and Behavioural Instability Phase

By this stage, physical changes in the brain may erode emotional self-control and judgment as well as the ability to interpret and solve problems, to handle stress, and to communicate verbally. Loved ones may start to express their fears and distress with uninhibited emotions and behaviours, such as anger and aggression. This can be the most stressful and emotionally draining phase for both caregiver and care receiver, although not everyone with dementia will display uncharacteristic behaviours.

A person at this stage isn't as aware of their disease as they were in the early stage; however, they usually still know something is wrong with them, but they can't quite put their finger on it. By the end of this phase, a person likely will have difficulty handling their personal care and walking without assistance. This happens when they are unable to make their body do familiar tasks and may have lost their sense of balance.

A summary follows of the symptoms in each area of decline for the middle stage of Alzheimer's disease.

Middle Stage: Emotional and Behavioural Instability Phase

Areas of Decline	Symptoms that May Occur
Cognitive Deficits	**Memory** • Declining recollection of recent events and personal history • Forgetting purpose of common utensils, such as a fork or toothbrush • Inability to recognize some or most family and friends **Communications** • Repeating words, reduced vocabulary, down to short sentences and yes or no answers • Difficultly organizing words logically • Declining ability to read, write, and understand people

	Reasoning
	• Difficulty with complex tasks, such as finances and choosing clothes • Declining ability to concentrate and often confused • Disorientation about time and place
Mood & Emotions	• Mood swings ranging from frustration, anxiety, apprehension, anger, hostility and fear, to sadness, depression, and crying • Feeling of helplessness
Uncharacteristic Behaviour	• Pleading to go home when in an unfamiliar environment • Withdrawn in socially or mentally challenging situations • Restlessness, pacing, or wandering may occur when feeling anxious • Repeating words, questions, or actions • Stressed out or anxious • Psychosis, such as hallucinations, delusions, paranoia, suspiciousness, hoarding, or stealing when misinterpreting what is seen or heard • Agitated or aggressive, such as shouting, name calling, or swearing when person is feeling angry, frustrated, or upset. • Catastrophic reactions, sudden fits of rage or combativeness, such as pinching, hitting, kicking, or biting, may be reaction to stress, being upset, or restrained • Uninhibited or sexual behaviour • Fearing a bath
Physical Problems	• Difficulty handling personal care and walking, at higher risk of falling • Disrupted sleep patterns and appetite fluctuations • May become incontinent • Visual perception problems (e.g., not able to orient utensils and small objects for correct use)

It was a really awful moment for me when I realized that my mother no longer knew who I was and I often drove back to Toronto during that middle stage with tears in my eyes. I was saddened and felt helpless as I witnessed my mother's ever-deteriorating mental state. I grieved the loss of our close relationship. It was tough on David too. On one of his visits Mom defiantly told him that he was not her son.

Thankfully, my melancholy soon evaporated. One day when I visited my mother, a registered practical nurse said to Doris in a cheery voice, "Your daughter is here to see you." Mom replied with a pleased look of surprise, "Oh for heaven's sake." The nurse and I both burst out laughing because we discovered that Doris, with her witty one-liners, was still with us.

Late Stage: The Docile Phase

I describe the late stage as docile because people who have reached this juncture usually can only utter the odd word or phrase. Their emotional and behavioural expressions of fear and distress usually have mellowed by then. They also sleep longer and more often and usually can't initiate any activities. Loved ones may appear to withdraw into their own world. However, they likely are still very aware and comforted by the presence and gentle touch of family and friends.

I used to think that people didn't die from Alzheimer's disease, but from some other ailment. I have since learned that dementia can make elders more vulnerable to infections and trigger the body to start to shut down. The three most common causes of death are as follows:

- Pneumonia: a person becomes so sedentary that they lose their ability to cough and clear their lungs.
- Stopping to eat or drink: a person loses their automatic reflex to chew and swallow.
- Pulmonary aspiration: a person loses their ability to cough up food and fluids that can get into their windpipe and lungs.

A summary of the symptoms that may occur in this late stage are listed on the next page.

Late Stage: The Docile Phase

Areas of Decline	Symptoms that May Occur
Cognitive Deficits	**Memory** • No longer recognizes family or friends • Loss of both short- and long-term memory **Communications** • Vocabulary declines to single words or a phrase and unrecognizable chatter, eventually losing ability to speak • Using non-verbal communications, facial expressions, body language, crying, grunting or groaning sounds • Lose ability to read and write **Reasoning** • Severe disorientation about time, place, and people • Ability to process information is severely impaired • Can no longer initiate activities
Mood & Emotions	• Become docile and withdrawn
Uncharacteristic Behaviour	• Repeating motions • Fascinated with small objects and may try to eat non-food items • May confuse a waste paper basket for a toilet
Physical Problems	• Sleeping longer and more often • Lose ability to walk without assistance • Eventually need support to sit • Lose ability to smile and hold head up • Usually need help eating and has difficulty chewing, drinking, and swallowing, resulting in weight loss • Reduced visual field, so may only see straight ahead • Joint and muscle rigidity may make putting on clothes difficult • Decreasing ability to use toilet, become incontinent • Immune system becomes weaker, increasing risk of infections • At end of life, may lose automatic reflex to swallow or cough

In the late stage, I became more accepting of my mother's illness, although I found it strange to call my mother Doris when I greeted her and to introduce myself as Shirley, her daughter. Her vocabulary had declined to mostly one or two words, such as, "Oh boy," if she was in discomfort or anxious, and, "Yeah," as a positive response to a question. I would have given anything to have back the many phone calls I received most days from my mother when she lived alone and first moved into a retirement residence.

LEARN CAREGIVING STRATEGIES FOR A HIGHER QUALITY OF LIFE TOGETHER

Dealing with dementia was at times emotionally draining, filling me with feelings of impatience, guilt, and sadness. Surprisingly though, spending five years visiting my mother in an Alzheimer's unit of a nursing home was an unforgettably positive experience for me. I discovered the joy and soothing calm of laughter that comes from interacting with residents who at times showed their devilish, charming, or amusing characters, despite their many disabilities.

I grew quite attached to some of the residents. One day, I observed that a silver-haired jolly man would throw the personal support workers a kiss. I got into the habit of giving him a big smile and throwing him a kiss whenever I saw him. When I did, he would grin from ear to ear, and then throw me back a kiss as he chuckled.

Alzheimer's disease has taught me that people are so much more than their collected memories. I am amazed and delighted that despite the ever-creeping destruction of brain cells, the human spirit is so very resilient. While our loved ones may no longer remember who we are, we don't lose the person they were before they developed the disorder.

Even in the last phase of the disease my mother never let me forget her personhood. In the middle of lunch one day, a pretty woman in her early 70s repeatedly said to my mother and me, "I'm going, I'm going." Doris lost her patience because she had heard this every mealtime for several weeks. After days of barely uttering a word, Mom leaned forward, looked the woman straight in the eye, and boldly said to her, "Then go!" I couldn't hold back my laughter and my tears of joy in hearing from my tenacious mother once again.

People living with Alzheimer's disease have the same range of emotions and likes and dislikes as the rest of us, and can respond to the emotions of others. Their personhood remains intact regardless of the stage of the disease. They still enjoy affection and can feel joy, love, and happiness, as well as fear, anxiety, anger, stress, frustrations, depression, and sadness.

Unfortunately, these lovable people do lose their ability to manage their own well-being. Their quality of life becomes dependent upon the quality of care they receive from caregivers, and their interactions and relationships with others. With information adapted from the Alzheimer Society as well as my own insights, I will share caregiver strategies that helped me reduce my stress level, take better care of my mother, and enjoy our life together.

Learn New Ways to Communicate

As people with Alzheimer's disease gradually lose their ability to speak and understand other people, their family will need to learn new ways to communicate with them. Families should speak in a calm, cheerful tone of voice to help ensure their message is well received. Messages should be positive in nature. For instance, instead of saying "don't go there" say, "let's go here." Voice pitch should be low and clear, and tempo should be slow and deliberate to maximize comprehension.

Getting the attention of a person with dementia and making eye contact will also help in the message delivery, as well as using short, simple sentences that contain familiar words. Delivering one concise message at a time will allow a loved one to follow a conversation.

If verbal messages do not appear to be understood, then combining words with gestures and visual cues usually helps, such as pointing to the door when asking if they want to go outside for a walk. Always assume, however, that a person with dementia can understand you. Never stop talking to your loved one, even if they can no longer speak. If you do, you could miss out on meaningful conversations on their good days.

Orienting information should be provided when a loved one no longer knows a family member, friend, or health-care provider. Everyone should greet a person in the middle and late stages of dementia by introducing themselves and calling them by their name. Then, if there are any caregiving tasks to do, such as brushing their hair or teeth, caregivers should first explain what they propose doing before proceeding.

It is important to continue to express your love in a manner that is comfortable and familiar to both you and your loved one. For Mom, hugs, kisses, and holding her hand always made her happy.

When trying to understand what a person with dementia is saying, caregivers need to be patient listeners and not correct them. In the first stage of the disease, my mother often asked me the same question repeatedly. With time, I learned to answer repeated questions as if they were the first time I heard them. It is a good idea to let other care providers know the names of important people and places in your loved one's life, so they may be better able to understand what your parent or spouse is talking about.

When you can't understand your loved one, try to make sense of the spoken words or phrases and respond to the emotional tone of the statement, by saying for example, "You seem to be angry," or "You seem to be sad." Their expressed feelings are more accurate than what they are saying.

When a person can't speak any longer, watch their eyes, facial expressions, gestures, actions, and other body language, and any sounds they make as an indication of how they are feeling, or reacting to other people and their environment.

My mother spoke with her big brown eyes. They would sparkle when we greeted her if she recognized a familiar face. A frown and a grimace meant she was in pain or uncomfortable. She would stare in fascination at children and pets and sometimes when someone read to her, if she wasn't too tired. Mom also spoke with her hands. She would hold tightly onto a hand, once offered, to express her affection.

Learn to Prevent or Resolve Defensive and Responsive Behaviours

Learning how to deal with what appeared to be my mother's seemingly inappropriate and irrational behaviour was one of the toughest challenges that I faced. I vividly remember my torment one afternoon two years after my father died. My mother asked me where my father was. I reminded her that he had died. She was devastated. In an uncharacteristic fit of rage she shouted, "Why didn't you tell me?"

In shock and with a feeling of a young child being scolded, I had no reply to offer. With time, I learned to not take this behaviour personally. Instead, I put myself in my mother's shoes and tried to understand the new world she lived in from her perspective, and with her disabilities. I realized that Mom had forgotten that Dad had died and wanted to know where he was, because at that moment she was feeling anxious.

I used a technique called "sidestepping" to redirect her thinking. I found a calming response, which was, "Dad is fine. He is in Cobourg and is busy doing chores around the house." That answer always pleased and reassured my mother that everything was fine. She would immediately drop the subject and go back to whatever she was doing. I got her caregiver-companions and personal support workers to use the same response when she asked that question.

Caregivers may at first feel hurt by anger directed at them, and mistakenly think the personality of their parent or spouse has changed. From time to time, we would all like to yell at someone when we feel we have been wronged; however, unlike people living with Alzheimer's disease, our emotional self-control is still intact. We usually refrain from lashing out and are capable of finding a more appropriate way to get our point across.

While there may not be an obvious reason for inappropriate behaviour, there is usually a cause for a sudden flare up of aggression, anxiety, or combativeness in a person with Alzheimer's disease. A defensive behaviour, such as hitting, kicking, or pinching is sometimes the only way a person with this disorder can protect themselves, or try to maintain some sense of control in their life. Combativeness might be triggered by being restrained or having a fear of certain activities, such as taking a bath.

Feelings of anxiety, confusion, or stress might trigger a responsive behaviour, such as pacing or wandering. Pleading to go home is another common responsive behaviour that might be triggered by being in a place unfamiliar or uncomfortable to them.

With great regularity in the first six months that Doris lived in the nursing home she pleaded with me to take her home. This always tugged at my heartstrings. I discovered after tremendous anguish that home in my mother's mind was with her parents in her childhood home in Lamaline, where she felt loved and secure. It wouldn't have mattered if Doris were back in her house in Cobourg or not, her brain couldn't recognize where she was at that particular moment.

I used sidestepping to get my mother to shift gears mentally by saying, "Mom, you must really miss your home. It was a very comfortable home." Those words always made her feel safe so she would stop asking to go home.

Through trial and error, there is often a way for caregivers to prevent or resolve inappropriate behaviours. The key is to learn the triggers of defensive and responsive behaviours that are specific to each individual and what works best for them. I discovered other ways of diffusing defensive and responsive behaviours that I learned from the Alzheimer Society and the staff in Mom's nursing home.

- Learn the warning signals that a person's stress level is rising and stop whatever you are doing. *No* always means *no*.
- Use humour, gentle cajoling, and cheerfulness to get a person to do something they don't want to do.
- Don't be bossy or condescending, or ignore the person.

- Don't react to verbal outbursts with your own anger. Saying "I am sorry" sometimes helps. Other times, leaving and coming back a few minutes later works.

- Learn to be creative. For example, disguise doors with paint or wallpaper to prevent wandering.

- Avoid asking too many questions over a short period of time.

- Don't argue or try to reason with the person. Go along with their perception of reality. Use sidestepping technique to redirect or distract a person, and reassure them everything will be fine. A hug may also help.

- Keep the environment as quiet, uncrowded, and calm as you can and the temperature comfortable.

- Don't get upset or offended by behaviour directed at you.

You won't always be able to prevent or resolve defensive behaviour, but you can learn from your mistakes, as I did. It is important to remind yourself that you are doing the best you can.

Meet Special Health-Care Needs

Providing medical care to people with Alzheimer's disease when they get sick or injured is more difficult than for other people, for a number of reasons. First, they usually are unable to complain if they are in pain, say that they feel ill, or explain why they aren't eating or drinking well. Second, when they receive medical treatment they may respond with defensive behaviour because they are frightened. This could limit the care they receive. Third, rehabilitation can be difficult because they lack the initiative and memory to repeat physiotherapy exercises on their own. Fourth, hospitalization may lead to a more rapid mental and physical decline.

Caregivers should tune into how their loved one uniquely expresses their feelings, level of comfort, distress, and pain. Even if they can no longer communicate well, there are obvious signs of discomfort or pain to look for, such as a tense or grimacing face, repeated words or groans, or guarding of a particular area of their body. Caregivers should alert medical professionals when they see signs of this type of behaviour.

A hospital filled with unfamiliar sights, sounds, odours, and hustle and bustle can cause fear, confusion, anxiety, and agitation in people living with Alzheimer's disease. For any medical appointment or procedure it is best to accompany a person with Alzheimer's disease. If they have to stay in the hospital then they need as many visitors as you can muster.

Caregivers can go through a great deal of anguish when their loved one does not eat well. I know I certainly did. A physical problem may be affecting their eating habits. The cause could be constipation, a stomach problem, a new medication, or a medical illness, such as a heart condition, diabetes, or depression. The reason could also be something very simple. According to a First Link coordinator with the Alzheimer Society of Kingston, when the eyeglasses of residents in a particular nursing home were cleaned the amount they ate increased.

Poor teeth, sore gums, or ill-fitting dentures can also affect the ability and willingness to eat. People with dementia often forget to brush their teeth, or lose their ability to use a toothbrush. Furthermore, they may dislike having their teeth brushed by someone else, so they commonly have teeth problems.

To solve this problem, Sharon, one of Mom's caregiver-companions, tried using children's fruit-flavoured toothpaste and a child's toothbrush. That worked very well, but, regrettably, our teeth-brushing discipline came too late. My mother developed infected roots from teeth that had fallen out and she required dental surgery to remove them. That turned out to be a problem, because when David took Mom to see a dentist she refused to open her mouth.

After that, I successfully lobbied the director of care in Mom's nursing home to bring in a dementia-friendly dental service for all residents on a regular basis. Shortly thereafter, a dentist was able to remove one infected root of a tooth. However, when he came back for my mother's second extraction, after freezing her mouth, she lurched forward and spit at him, in a defensive response. The dentist recoiled and refused to go further. I quickly found a dementia-friendly oral surgeon who removed Mom's remaining infected roots while she was sedated in a hospital.

Mom could have died from the infection if it had gotten into her bloodstream or from malnutrition, because in four years her weight had plummeted from 49 to 33 kilograms (108 to 70 pounds). Her gums became so sore that she resisted eating. Fortunately, Mom's weight returned to normal within a year, which was perfect for her petite five-foot-one frame.

In the late stage of the disease, elders often need assistance to eat their meals. They have more difficulty chewing, drinking, and swallowing, can't remember how to eat anymore or whether they ate or not. They usually need to be sitting upright and eating in a quiet environment without too many distractions. Offering bite-sized pieces of food that can be picked up with fingers often helps. However, loved ones may need pureed food, and thickened soups and beverages, to prevent them from choking. This is a particular concern because in late-stage Alzheimer's disease they are likely to lose their automatic reflex to swallow and cough up secretions.

It is a good idea to keep an extra set of eyeglasses and hearing aids on hand, because people with dementia tend to lose them. Their names should be put on these assistive devices, and their optometrist and audiologist should keep their prescription for eyeglasses and hearing aid moulds respectively. Another reason is because their eyesight and hearing can no longer be tested once they reach the middle stage of Alzheimer's disease. By then, their cognitive skills will have declined and they won't be able to answer complex questions.

Help Elders Feel Comfortable and Safe

People living with Alzheimer's disease have higher needs to feel safe and comfortable than the rest of us, as they struggle to make sense of what is wrong with them. They respond best to familiar people, the same daily routine and to an environment that is familiar, free from the distractions of crowds and loud noises, and a comfortable temperature.

Visits from family and friends, even though they may not be recognized or remembered, provide stimulation and comfort. While visiting, however, it is important to not exhibit any negative emotions or facial expressions of anger, impatience, or frustration.

A person with Alzheimer's disease assimilates emotions very easily and may feel hurt if emotions are directed at them.

Encourage Independence and Boost Self-Esteem

A person living with dementia may feel devalued if their friends or family treat them as if they are no longer there, talk about them in front of them, or treat them as a child. It is best not to fall into this hurtful habit because they are usually more aware than they appear. Make them feel valued, useful, and independent by focusing on what they can still do, rather than what they can no longer do.

A person with dementia will feel more independent if they are given the ability to make as many decisions as they are capable of making. To do that, caregivers may need to reduce the number of choices they offer, such as picking between two meal options or activities. Mom's caregiver-companions often asked her to pick what clothes she wanted to wear the next day.

It is also best to ask for yes or no answers whenever possible, rather than asking complex questions that rely on a good memory. As well, breaking tasks and hobbies down into simple familiar steps, and providing step-by-step guidance, such as "unbutton your pyjama top, then take it off," rather than "get undressed" usually works better.

Making a loved one feel involved and useful will build their self-esteem. This can be accomplished by asking them to help you do small household tasks, such as folding laundry or setting the table for dinner in the early and middle stages, or by holding a book for you to read in the late stage. Giving them praise and encouragement as they work will also lift their spirits, as it will do for any of us.

Enjoy Activities Together

Caregivers and care receivers can have a better quality of life if they continue to share their favourite passions in life. Finding opportunities to laugh and have fun will lighten the load of dementia for both of you.

Engage a spouse or parent in activities that they enjoy and want to participate in, and that stimulate their mind. There should be, however, an appropriate level of challenge and assistance for their level of capability. Reading a story, a poem, a religious book, or a magazine to a loved one can be an enjoyable pastime. Even without words to share, sharing silence by sitting peacefully beside a beautiful garden can provide many pleasurable moments together.

Caregivers can stay connected with their parent or spouse by stimulating their sensory perceptions. Their primary senses of touching, hearing, tasting, and smelling usually remain intact, and while they may have tunnel vision they can still see. People with dementia can seem to be frozen in time in the middle and late stages. Surprisingly, the sound of music can magically bring them to a state of alertness, and provide comfort and familiarity, if it is music that they relate to from their past.

When Mom was in the late stage, the small activities room in the Alzheimer's unit of her nursing home was converted into a Snoezelen Multi-Sensory Environment. These recreational therapy rooms are designed for people with sensory impairment or neurological disorders. They stimulate the senses with combinations of music, interesting sounds, lighting effects, movement, gentle vibrations, tactile sensations, aromatherapy, and lots of colour. The room relaxes people with dementia and gives them a focal point. Participants and caregivers can improve their communications in this fun yet calming recreational atmosphere.

The moving stars in a galaxy that were projected on the ceiling in the darkened room particularly fascinated my mother. She also liked the colourful bubbles that streamed and rose in a water bubble tube, and the sound of a toy dolphin as it gently moved up and down on a pedestal when plugged in. Mom and I both enjoyed the scent of lavender essential oil, which is known for its relaxing aroma.

This unique multi-sensory environment stirred Mom to a calm state of alertness. The room woke up my senses too. We were having fun together once again, as we did when I was a little girl. I found real joy in helping my mother to have as full a life as she could have at this stage. Families can find out more information about Snoezelen Rooms and the techniques and tools used by visiting http://snoezeleninfo.com.

While I learned many lessons about caring for a person with dementia one of the most important was to slow down and live in the moment, as they do. I realized my mother wouldn't always be with me so I grew to appreciate every day we spent together and to express my love to her often. It didn't matter that she no longer knew who I was. She was my beloved mother, who still had feelings and loved to be loved.

TOP TIPS

Caregiving Is the Primary Treatment for Dementia

- People living with dementia eventually lose their ability to manage their own well-being.
- Their quality of life becomes dependent upon the quality of care they receive from caregivers, and their interactions and relationships with others.

An Early Diagnosis Is Very Important

- Medications designed to slow disease progression work best when taken in the early stages of Alzheimer's disease.
- The person and their family will have time to plan for the type of care that will be needed and to prepare emotionally for what lies ahead.

Gain an Understanding of Disease Progression

- Learn about the three stages of Alzheimer's disease:
  - Early stage: Period of disease awareness and frustration

○ Middle stage: Emotional and behavioural instability phase

○ Late stage: Docile phase

People with Alzheimer's Disease Never Lose their Personhood

- They retain their full range of emotions. They can enjoy affection and can feel love and happiness, as well as fear, anger, and sadness.

- Their primary senses of touching, seeing, hearing, tasting, and smelling remain intact.

Learn to Communicate in New Ways

- Speaking slowly, calmly, and in a cheerful tone of voice will help ensure your message is understood and well received.

- Be a patient listener and don't correct your parent or spouse.

- Combine words with gestures and visual cues when messages do not appear to be understood.

- Your loved one's expressed feelings are more accurate than what they are saying.

Try to Prevent or Resolve Defensive Behaviours

- Put yourself in the shoes of your spouse or parent, and see the world from their perspective and disabilities.

- Look for underlying cause of defensive behaviours, and through trial and error, find the best techniques to prevent or diffuse them.

- Don't get upset or offended by behaviours directed at you.

(Continued)

Meet Special Health-Care Needs

- Read signs of discomfort or pain and alert medical professionals if needed.
- Accompany your loved one to medical appointments. Don't leave them alone for long in hospitals without as many visitors as you can muster.
- Don't forget to take care of their teeth.
- Uncover causes of eating problems.
- Keep extra set of glasses and hearing aids because they tend to lose them.

Help Elders Feel More Comfortable and Safe

- As best you can, keep everything familiar—people, routines, and environment.
- Don't show negative emotions or facial expressions.

Encourage Independence and Boost Self-Esteem

- Make loved ones feel involved and useful by having them help with small tasks.
- Break tasks into small steps.
- Let loved ones participate in decisions by giving them a few choices.
- Ask for yes or no answers rather than asking complex questions.
- Offer praise and encouragement.
- Don't fall into hurtful habits of treating parent or spouse as if they are no longer there, or talk about them in front of them, or treat them as a child.

Enjoy Activities Together

- Share favourite passions in life and find opportunities to laugh and have fun.
- Use music to comfort and add familiarity.
- Share silence when there are no longer any words to share.
- Awaken primary senses to find a fun way to connect with loved one in late stage.

(12)

The Last Life of Doris

The grace, balance, and agility of cats that allows them to land on their feet when falling from great heights may be behind the ancient legend that cats have nine lives. Doris had this feline resiliency and five times she avoided death by just a whisker.

At seven, she survived scarlet fever and four years later, a tsunami hit Lamaline, but Doris, her family, and their house were spared. When she was 17, suffering from severe abdominal pain and a fever, her parents transported her by horse-drawn boxcart to the nearest hospital in Grand Bank, 40 kilometres away, where an obstructed bowel was cleared just in time. When Doris turned 80 her hardy genes, a deep faith in God, and a strong will to live, helped her survive post-operative complications from having a pacemaker implanted. Five years later, she cheated death one last time when a blood clot formed in her leg after surgery. If the clot had broken loose and travelled to her lung she could have died from a pulmonary embolism.

The last six years of my mother's life proved to be very challenging for her, but even in the middle stage of Alzheimer's disease she made visitors feel welcomed and appreciated. She gave them a radiant smile, and when she was able, she thanked them for coming and asked if they would come again. She even found ways to express her love, by holding on to my hand, and the hands of her caregiver-companions. Doris still had an abundance of love to share with her family and friends.

In the summer of 2007 when Mom was 89, the battery life of her pacemaker needed to be replaced. Since she almost died putting the pacemaker in eight years earlier, David and I agonized over the decision of whether to have the battery replaced or not. Medical decisions are always difficult when a loved one has become incapacitated, and is in a life-threatening situation with no hope of recovery or resumption of a normal independent life. This crisis made us realize that we should have talked to our parents about their end-of-life wishes when they were much younger.

We would likely have had a very general discussion about under what circumstances they would choose medical intervention, and when they would not. For instance, we might have talked about whether they wanted to be resuscitated from a heart attack if they had terminal cancer, or whether they wanted a mechanical ventilator to breathe for them if they had a stroke and were permanently paralyzed.

It would have been very helpful to know Mom's response to these more general questions. Instead, we were in the gut-wrenching position of choosing life or death for another human being without their input. However, even if we *had* had that discussion and knew their wishes, this decision would still be tough to make because substitute decision-makers have to interpret those wishes for the specific situation. Then they must give medical professionals an informed consent or refusal of consent to treatment.

Fortunately, David and I had the availability of time for discussions with specialists to help us make this anguished but calm decision, because the battery life of Mom's pacemaker was not expected to run out for about three to five months. In contrast, family caregivers are often required to make decisions at lightning speed in hospital ER and intensive care units. Understanding a loved one's wishes becomes even more helpful under those circumstances.

We sought the advice of Mom's cardiologist, two family doctors, the nursing-home administrator, and a social worker. The cardiologist said he thought the risks of the surgery significantly outweighed the benefits, because Mom was not very dependent upon the pacemaker, using it only 0 to 5 per cent of the time.

Furthermore, the plastic around the lead wire of the pacemaker might be so brittle that it would have to be replaced, which could lead to yet another punctured lung. There was also a risk of infection from the incision, a common danger with any surgery, and a greater threat to the elderly of contracting a hospital virus.

Michael, my friend who is a family physician, said, "Replacing the pacemaker battery would be artificially keeping your mother alive. It's time for God to take her home." I embarrassingly broke down in tears, but I knew I had received good heartfelt advice.

The social worker offered many pearls of wisdom to help us make our decision. I began by asking her a question that had been nagging my brother and me: "How do we live with our decision if we make the wrong one?" She said there is no wrong decision at the last stage of life because my mother's health would only get worse. She went on to say, "As a society we keep people alive just because we can, but we must think about quality versus length of life." She had elderly clients who spoke about when it was their time to go, and would often say, "Just let God take me when it's my time."

The woman then asked me if I were in my mother's shoes what I thought she would have wanted. My answer was to not go ahead with the surgery, because Doris had reached the late stage of Alzheimer's disease. She was totally dependent upon others for all activities of daily living and was sleeping more often.

The social worker left me with a lot to think about, "Your anguish over your decision shows how caring you are," she said "but also that you don't want to let go." I realized the truth in her words, and that saying goodbye to my mother would be difficult to do, but inevitable.

David and I decided to not replace the pacemaker battery and "to let her be and let nature take its course," as her wise and compassionate family doctor had suggested. The decision-making process had been a growing experience about love, life, and letting go.

As it turned out, Doris went on to live another two years and heart failure was not the cause of her death. She had no further fainting spells as she had before the pacemaker was put in, so replacing the pacemaker battery would have put her through unnecessary surgery with all the associated risks.

On September 8, 2008, I held a luncheon party to celebrate my mother's 90th birthday. Fourteen kind-hearted ladies who had all made a difference in Mom's life attended, including Gladys, Doris' 96-year-old sister, and her niece who came from Ottawa for the festivities. Doris slept through most of her birthday celebration, except when it was time to eat birthday cake.

By then, Doris seldom spoke, except for a few words now and then, and unrecognizable chatter. She no longer savoured food with pleasure as she once had, and at times needed to have her cheek massaged to remind her to swallow. Every time I noticed a decline in my mother's health I felt death's door open a little wider.

In our society, death is considered an unfriendly intruder. We may accept the cycle of life as long as it happens to someone else, but oftentimes not to us personally or to our family. Funerals are the one family event that we anticipate the least and for which we are unprepared.

Let's face it. Most of us have our heads in the sand when it comes to the *d* word. We are afraid of dying, of excruciating pain, and of being alone when we leave this earth. Many adults are even in denial of their own mortality because medical advances are keeping their parents alive for so very long.

I learned an important lesson about death from Susan, a friend who was a former consulting client. She spent a year reading everything she could find about life and death when she was going through chemo and radiation therapy for breast cancer. "Our culture doesn't allow us to accept physical decline and dying," she said, "so we go through tremendous anguish when they occur." Hollywood has created such an appetite for fantasy and happy endings that we are uncomfortable with more realistic portrayals.

She also said, "We are control freaks." We have a script in our heads of how our life will unfold and we avoid thinking or talking about our own mortality and that of our loved ones. Susan thinks we need to learn to let go, to accept that we don't have control over when our loved ones and we will die.

I used to think, as a caregiver, that I had to control everything in my mother's life, but then I realized she was a child of God, and she was in His waiting room. It was my job to keep her as comfortable and happy as I could while she was still with us, but it was up to God to decide when it was her time to go. This understanding gave me a sense of inner peace.

By the spring of 2009, Doris' body and organs were showing signs of exhaustion, but, surprisingly, she was still with us. She slept peacefully most of the time, no longer spoke, and seldom even uttered a sound. Eating was becoming more difficult for her because she was losing her ability to swallow. She lost eight pounds over the winter.

By mid-August 2009, I started to make plans for Mom's 91st birthday in September. On Tuesday, August 18, Mitch and I left for the cottage for a week's holiday. Just as we arrived, I received a call from a registered nurse in my mother's nursing home telling me that my mother had just been put on oxygen because her breathing had become laboured. The nurse suspected that food or fluids had gotten into Mom's windpipe and lungs and blocked her wind passage, a condition called pulmonary aspiration, which occurred because her automatic reflex to chew, swallow, and cough up secretions had been destroyed.

Realizing the seriousness of her condition, several caregiver-companions stayed with her into the evening. Because she was having difficulty breathing, Eleanor decided to spend the night to lower Mom's anxiety level. I called David, who was on vacation in France, to let him know of this new development. His flight back to Vancouver was booked for the following Monday. I also stayed in touch with the registered nurse and registered practical nurse on duty that night and the next day. They weren't sure whether Mom would stabilize or get worse, so they said they didn't know whether I should come home or not.

Later the next day, she was taken off oxygen because her O2 level had returned to normal. Her colour was better too, and she was able to swallow a small amount of thickened water and a nutritional supplement. On Thursday, Mitch and I decided to drive home from our cottage in Quebec. If Mom was sick, I needed to be with her. I was back in the nursing home by Friday morning and relieved that I was because she took a turn for the worse.

She was hot and clammy and still not eating or drinking much. She was very sleepy and her pulse was abnormally low, at 34 beats per minute (normal for an adult is between 50 and 80). It was at that juncture that I made the decision to start a vigil with Mom's caregiver-companions, the nursing staff, and myself by her side that lasted for little more than a week.

Mom looked worn out and more lifeless than I had ever seen her before. As sadness filled my heart, I realized it was time for her to go. When I got home later that day I went for a walk in the tiny town of Bath on the shore of Lake Ontario near Kingston, where Mitch and I had retired the previous summer. I always find that walking gives me solace during troubling times.

I walked past St. John's Anglican Church, the charming little place of worship established in 1787 that I had joined. It was six o'clock on a Friday evening, so I didn't know why I tried to open the front door, because it should have been locked, but I did. Surprisingly, it opened and I entered, walking slowly toward the darkened pews and the well-lit altar. I had the church all to myself. With tears trickling down my face, I prayed that Mom would be taken to heaven soon, without suffering any pain. Until that moment, I had prayed only that He take her when He was ready. It seemed as if I was meant to have this private time with God.

I felt it was vitally important for me to meet Mom's spiritual needs in this final chapter of her life, because her Christian faith had been such a big part of the person she was. I called Pauline, her good friend, who was in charge of pastoral care for Mom's church and who had visited her regularly over the past seven years. I asked if she and Father Peter could visit my mother and say a prayer for her.

Pauline came the very next day, on Saturday, August 22. She recited a prayer and asked Mom, "Doris, do you want to go to heaven to be with God and your husband, Ed?" Surprisingly, Mom blinked her eyes very noticeably. I'm not sure whether she heard and understood the question and was responding in the affirmative in the only way she could express herself, but I would like to think that she did.

Sensing that she needed to hear these words from me, I said, "Mom, it's okay for you to go now. David and I will miss you very much, but we will be fine on our own now." I hoped that my assurances would give her closure on her life here on Earth, so that she would be ready to depart.

Mitch and I spent Sunday with Mom. We took her out to the courtyard where she could enjoy the gardens and the beautiful sunny day. There was a refreshing breeze coming in off Lake Ontario that made the temperature as perfect as a summer day could be. She had much better colour and her breathing seemed normal, so unrealistically I was still hopeful that she would stabilize.

On Monday, August 24, my mother's priest, Canon Peter Walker, anointed her and gave her a blessing, commending her to God's eternal care. The parish nurse said healing prayers asking for God's blessing for her body, mind, and spirit, and comfort for her family. Peter and Diane were well schooled in leaving a notation in Doris' visitor book, and I was pleased that this time was no exception.

Surprisingly, the next morning, Doris II, another one of Mom's caregiver-companions, reported with great delight that Mom started to eat again. She had some oatmeal, half a glass of nutritional supplement, and a few spoonfuls each of yogurt, pureed toast, thickened orange juice, and water. We all thought that finally she was starting to recover. Our hopes, however, were soon dashed. By lunchtime, Mom only took five small spoonfuls of water and would not swallow. She showed no interest in eating or drinking at dinnertime either, even though it had been a full week since she ate normally.

Eating and drinking typically taper off in people as the dying process begins. The body no longer needs energy so they don't desire food or feel hunger as their digestive system slows down. Kidneys start to shut down once fluids are no longer passing through them. Mom developed a fever at that point, so the nurses started to administer Tylenol suppositories on a regular basis to lower her temperature and keep her comfortable.

That same day, Eleanor discovered clumps of thick mucus at the back of my mother's mouth and throat, an indication of respiratory congestion and that death was drawing near. She was able to remove some of the mucus by using a glycerine swab. Respiratory congestion occurs when the ability to swallow and cough weakens, the production of saliva and bronchial mucous secretions increase in the throat and airway, the airway diameter decreases from swelling, or breathing patterns change.

Our care team went into high-gear palliative-care mode. Doris' caregiver-companions worked longer hours and gathered around her even when they were not on duty, so that she would not be alone, and would be as comfortable as they could make her. The nurses were also very attentive and in communication with Doris' doctor, to ensure she had the right medications to manage her pain and keep her comfortable. My mother had grown to trust these very familiar and compassionate health-care professionals, so she could rest at ease and die peacefully.

Two of the nurses on two separate occasions asked me if I wanted to send Doris to the hospital. I told them emphatically that the nursing home was my mother's home, and I wanted her to die at home. The choice of a place to die is extremely important. I couldn't recreate a Lamaline-style vigil in my parents' own home, but I could lovingly support my mother with a sisterhood of caregivers who knew, understood, and cared compassionately about her.

I didn't want Mom to spend her final days in an acute-care hospital where she would be very disoriented and stressed out by diagnostic tests, and electronic monitoring apparatus and machines; where the care is hurried, demanding, and impersonal, and focused on healing, not on dying. If a hospital has a palliative-care unit, however, that would be a better place to die than in a regular hospital ward. A palliative-care unit is not available in all hospitals though, and patients can, in most cases, only stay for a limited period of time. Furthermore, the unit can only be accessed if a patient obtains a doctors' referral, and there is a bed for him or her when needed.

I thought of calling a local hospice palliative-care agency for help, but I didn't think there was any need. If Mom hadn't had such attentive and compassionate care, then seeking hospice services would have been very welcomed support. At no cost to clients, hospice volunteers provide companionship to people living with a life-threatening or terminal illness. They also provide emotional support to clients and their families, respite for caregivers, spiritual support, and bereavement support. Hospice care can be administered collaboratively with other health-care providers in a patient's home, a hospital, retirement residence, or nursing home.

It would be preferable, though, to call in hospice when the terminal nature of a loved one's medical condition is first known. This could be as much as six months before they die. That way, the person can become familiar with the hospice volunteers and develop a trust in their care; however, even a few weeks of compassionate support can improve a dying person's emotional and physical comfort.

During my mother's vigil, I received support from one particular personal support worker who had just taken a palliative-care course. She taught me that death is a natural process that completes the life cycle and we shouldn't be afraid of it. I found her words very calming. I had been very stressed out wondering what would happen next and what more I could do for Mom. Later that day as I left for home, the director of care gave me a hug and a hospice palliative-care pamphlet to read to prepare me for Mom's approaching death.

I learned about Mom's comfort and care needs in her final days and hours from this pamphlet, the nursing staff in Mom's nursing home, Doris' caregiver-companions, and from a friend who is a registered nurse. I immediately put my learning into practice for Mom so that I could give her a good death.

Each person's death is very unique and it comes in its own time and way. When a death is expected at the end of a terminal illness, such as cancer, heart disease, ALS, Alzheimer's, or Parkinson's disease, there are similarities in the natural process of how our bodies shut down, which make it possible for us to plan for the care that will be needed. Something triggers the shutting down process of a body's systems when a person is already in a weakened state. In Mom's case it was pulmonary aspiration, which is common in late-stage Alzheimer's patients. In cancer and heart disease the trigger may be respiratory congestion, and for these and other illnesses it can be pneumonia, the flu, or some other assault on the body.

While there are many different causes of death, there are recognizable signs and symptoms that caregivers can look for that will indicate that the dying process has begun. Not all symptoms will be present though, and some may only appear in the last few minutes or hours of life. With this knowledge, caregivers can give their loved one the precious gift of a comfortable and peaceful death, by attending to their emotional, mental, and physical needs. I have included a Caregivers' Palliative-Care Guide in the Appendix on page 249 to help family caregivers prepare for this momentous time with their loved one.

During this participatory vigil, caregivers can stay connected with their loved one until the last moments of life, because in most cases they won't lose their emotions, sense of touch, or hearing until they lose consciousness. Even in a coma or semi-coma state, some palliative-care experts believe that patients can still be comforted by touch and talking.

Unknowingly, Mitch and I spent our very last day with my mother on Wednesday, August 26. She looked very peaceful, but she spent the day in bed because her pulse was low, at 37 beats per minute, and she was very clammy. When I read Doris' visitor book I noticed that a few of her caregiver-companions had written that as they held her hand she grasped their hand quite firmly, as she did mine. I knew then that my mother was very much aware of our presence, and that we were able to lift her spirits in her final hours.

Like David, I realize there are many other family members who will be unable to be with their loved one as death approaches. In this situation, it is important to connect by telephone with a parent or spouse if possible, and to have a meaningful conversation, and to say, "I love you." This parting exchange will help a loved one transcend into the afterlife more peacefully and, long after they have passed away, give family members a sense of peace as well.

My brother called our mother as soon as he returned to Vancouver from his holiday in France. Eleanor held the phone to her ear and I think Mom understood and appreciated what David was saying to her, because Eleanor noted in her visitor book, "Doris did move her eyes some when he spoke to her."

Before I left that day, I wrote in Doris' visitor book a number of palliative-care measures for Mom's caregiver-companions that Eleanor and I felt were needed:

- Hold her hand, and gently touch her to let her know she is not alone.
- Gently massage her heart, hands, and feet.
- Play her favourite hymns on her CD player.
- Reposition Mom about every 1 to 1½ hours, or 2 hours if she is in a deep sleep.
- Give her a sponge bath if she seems hot or clammy.
- Check her temperature, and if high, ask the registered practical nurse to give her a pain medication.
- Remove any mucus from her mouth and throat using a glycerine swab.
- Use glycerine swabs to alleviate dry mouth, and apply Vaseline to her lips to keep them moist.

I ended my notation with, "That should do it. Thanks everyone for your loving care."

By Thursday morning, Mom was not as comfortable. She seemed to be in some pain, was quite flushed and was coughing at times. The personal support workers, with the help of Mom's caregiver-companions, kept turning Mom and giving her a sponge bath. The registered practical nurses regularly gave her a medication for pain relief and the registered nurses kept a close watch. Alana, another one of Mom's caregiver-companions, read some lovely poems to her from *The Friendship Book,* and as she did, Doris' eyes were wide open and she was squeezing Alana's hand.

By that afternoon, Eleanor noticed Doris was experiencing slight tremors in her upper body so she knew the end was near. Alana came back to relieve Eleanor's lunch shift, and stayed with Mom until 10 p.m. Eleanor returned for the night shift.

She wanted to make sure that my mother was not alone in her final hours. By midnight, she noticed some mottling, which is blotchy purple-coloured skin, on Mom's hands and arms, as her blood circulation decreased.

Having cheated death five times over the course of her lifetime, God finally took Doris home on Friday, August 28. Coincidently, she died at exactly the same age as my Dad, just days before their 91st birthdays. My mother had a good life and she had a good death. Without any grimacing pain, and having been bedridden for only two days, she breathed her last laboured parting breath in the very early hours of Friday morning, at 1:20 a.m. She fleetingly opened her eyes to see Eleanor by her side, and to hear hymns playing in her own very familiar room in the nursing home. Eleanor's last entry in Doris' visitor book was:

1:00 a.m.

Turned Doris. A little more mottling.

Pulse 54. Strong, regular beat.

Swabbed mouth. Applied Vaseline to lips.

Massaged heart, hands, and feet.

Have played Doris' music softly all night.

1:15 a.m.

Doris stopped breathing and then took a laboured breath.

Rang for nurse. Personal support worker and nurse came.

1:20 a.m.

Doris stopped breathing.

The nurse and personal support worker were very good.

God bless, Doris. It has been a pleasure.

Doris' caregiver-companions and the nursing staff were all pros in palliative care. These kind-hearted women are truly the unsung heroes in our society because they dedicate their lives to caring for infirm elderly people, they grow very attached to these special souls, and then they gently and expertly shepherd them into the afterlife.

That Friday morning, I visited Mom in the funeral home in Cobourg, the same familiar place where I had taken Mom and Dad to make their funeral arrangements in 2001, and revisited just a year later for Dad's funeral. Mom looked so serene, as if the shackles of Alzheimer's disease had suddenly vacated her body. This was the first time I saw her mouth totally shut in over a year, and she looked to be a younger Doris. Apparently, when we go to heaven we leave our ailments behind us, so she must have made her way very quickly to the Pearly Gates. I'd like to think she is now living in eternal spring with her beloved Ed.

It is always a shock when someone dies, even if it is an expected death. It certainly was for me, when I was awakened at 1:30 a.m. that Friday morning by a registered nurse from Mom's nursing home with the news that Doris had breathed her last breath. I thought I would be well prepared and accepting of my mother's death. After all, I had been watching Mom's decline for seven years, and I finished writing her eulogy six months earlier. Instead, I felt as if I was a sailboat that had just come aground and lost the wind in its sails. I wasn't ready at all for the ground-swell of emotions that hit me, and the streams of tears that would gush down my face, sometimes at awkwardly telling moments, for many months afterwards.

I now understand that none of us is ever truly ready to lose our parents or our spouse. A friend comforted my bruised heart when she wrote in an e-mail to me, "As daughters, there is so much of our mothers in us—all the best things, I like to think. You will miss her terribly, but she lives on in and through you in large and small ways." I certainly hope that my mother's values and lively spirit will live on in me, as well as her deep compassion for others.

This book is a tribute to my mother, and has been a labour of love for very special elderly people who were once vibrant and strong, and who are now too ill to advocate for themselves. My hope is that the world will become a more compassionate place for them, where their physical, social, emotional, intellectual, and spiritual needs will attentively and lovingly be met. You and I will be them someday and we will want this type of quality care as well.

Doris holds a very special place in the hearts of all those who knew her. She had an optimistic attitude toward life that endeared her to her family and many close and lifelong friends. Her life's journey has been completed, but she has left us a legacy of valuable life lessons:

- Life is precious and should never be taken for granted.
- Believe in yourself, and you can do whatever you set your mind to.
- Share your love and kindness with the world.
- Look for the good in people for you will surely find it.
- Family is the most important priority in life.
- A strong faith in God can provide guidance and comfort during life's troubled waters.
- Be a good listener and focus more on other people than yourself.
- Remember to thank people for their acts of kindness toward you.
- There is no harm in asking. You will be amazed by what wishes will be granted.

One of my greatest joys in life has been the very close and loving relationship that I had with my mother. I truly miss her. If we listen carefully, though, perhaps we can hear people laughing at Doris' witty one-liners in heaven where she undoubtedly is.

TOP TIPS

Face Reality of Death Head On

- Accept inevitability of physical decline and dying, and the reality that we can't control when our loved ones and we will die.

Plan for Death

- Death is a natural process that completes the life cycle. We shouldn't be afraid of it, avoid thinking about it, or neglect planning for it.
- Prepare your own will, appoint a substitute decision-maker for personal care and property, and communicate care wishes. Encourage loved ones to do the same.

Prepare for Palliative-Care Needs

- Create a comfortable home or home-like setting for approaching death.
- Build palliative-care team early so loved one grows to trust these very familiar health-care specialists.

Give Precious Gift of a Peaceful Death

- Meet spiritual needs of loved one so they will transcend into the afterlife peacefully.
- Provide care that is compassionate, patient, and attentive to emotional, mental, and physical needs as the natural dying process shuts down the body.

Stay Connected until Last Moments of Life

- Most people will not lose their emotions, sense of touch, or hearing until the last moments of life.
- Stay connected by gently holding your loved one's hand, speaking calmly and clearly, and playing soft music to let him or her know they are not alone.

Appendix

CAREGIVERS' PALLIATIVE-CARE GUIDE

Emotional Changes and Comfort Needs

Signs & Symptoms of Approaching Death	Emotional Comfort Needed
Withdrawal	
• Withdrawal into own world, expressed by disinterest in people and surroundings. • Emotions are still intact. • Loved one may feel anxious.	• Gentle touch, holding hands, and hugging will demonstrate your love. • Speak with loving words. • Play soft music or sing songs with meaning to your loved one. • Read from their favourite books. • Use soft lighting, not too bright or dark. • Massage feet, hands, and heart regularly to calm patient and so they know someone is with them. • If necessary, ask nurse to order a sedative.

Mental Changes and Psychological Comfort Needs

Signs & Symptoms of Approaching Death	Psychological Comfort Needed
Disorientation & Restlessness	
• Medications, a decrease in oxygen to brain, and chemical changes in body can cause disorientation, restlessness, agitation, confusion, or inability to recognize familiar faces.	• Identify yourself by name. • Speak calmly and clearly. • Explain any care measures before starting.
Less Responsive then Unresponsive	
• Person sleeps much more. • Speaking decreases and eventually stops. • Person becomes unresponsive, even with eyes partially opened, and may eventually go into coma or semi-coma state.	• Continue care and speaking to loved one until breathing and heart stop.

Physical Changes and Care Needs

Signs & Symptoms of Approaching Death	Physical Care Needed
Decline then Cessation of Food & Liquid Intake	
• Food and liquids are not desired or needed as digestive system slows down. • Swallowing becomes more difficult or no longer possible. • Kidneys fail once liquids no longer pass through and a fever can develop. • Bowels eventually stop working. • Urine production declines and may be tea coloured.	• Don't force food or fluids. Offer small amounts of water or ice chips if person is alert and can still swallow. • Use lemon glycerine swabs regularly to alleviate dry mouth. • Put Vaseline on lips to keep them moist. • Ask attending physician to prescribe analgesic for pain, a bowel regime and a medication to reduce fever, and one to ease breathing.

Incontinence	
• As muscles relax person may lose control of urine or bowel matter.	• Check with physician to determine if catheter, or adult diapers are needed. • Keep loved one clean and comfortable.
Changes in Skin Temperature & Colour	

• As blood circulation decreases skin may become:
  ◦ cool and clammy, and very pale or waxy in appearance;
  ◦ mottled, blotchy, and purple-coloured on hands, arms, feet, or legs; or
  ◦ pale or bluish on the lips and under nails.
	• Give sponge bath and wipe forehead with a cool facecloth regularly.
	• Change bedding and pyjamas, as necessary.
	• Extra blankets are not necessary; they just add weight.

Limited Movement	
• Red or pink pressure points may appear on fragile skin as person becomes too weak to move or turn.	• Turn person every 1½ to 2 hours, using pillows to support them, and ensure they are in a comfortable position. • Ask nurse if massaging red spots on hips, shoulders, arms, and feet with lanolin cream will help to relieve discomfort and bring blood to area. • If skin starts to tear ask nurse to apply OpSite transparent polyurethane membrane, and to put a piece of lambswool under pressure points. If pressure points on feet, put in lambswool booties.

(Continued)

Signs & Symptoms of Approaching Death	Physical Care Needed
Respiratory Congestion	

• Respiratory congestion occurs when:
 	
  ○ cough reflex becomes ineffective;
  ○ production of saliva and bronchial mucous secretions increase in the throat and airway;
  ○ diameter of the airway decreases due to swelling; or
  ○ breathing patterns become more rapid.
	• Elevating head and putting person onto their side will encourage drainage, keep airway clear, and decrease pooling of secretions.
	• Ask nurse for medication patch that goes behind ear to dry up secretions.
	• Remove clumps of mucus and phlegm from the mouth and back of throat by using a glycerine swab.

Irregular Breathing Patterns	

• Decreasing circulation may cause irregular breathing patterns such as:
 	
  ○ Cheyne-Stokes: rapid breaths followed by pause in breathing, then regular breathing resumes
  ○ death rattle: noisy breathing because dying person unable to clear his or her throat
  ○ other abnormal patterns, such as laboured, shallow then deep, or slow then fast breathing
	• Raising head slightly and putting person onto their side may allow them to breathe more easily.
	• Keep the mouth moist and clean.
	• Ask nurse for medication to ease breathing at a time when energy is failing.

Senses May Be Dulled, but Hearing Still Present	
• Awareness of pain may decrease. • Sensitivity to touch remains. • Assume hearing still present even if loved one is unable to respond. • Vision may become blurred.	• Gently touching person when speaking to them will engage their senses and add comfort. • Continue with eye drops if person was accustomed to using them.

Index